"*SUPERWELL* is more than a book—it's a reflection of its author. Lauren, a Nutritious Life certified coach, is the poster child for what it means to thrive: living and breathing her passion, inspiring others, and embodying the very principles she teaches. In these pages, she offers a complete, practical, and inspiring guide to living your best life—one that proves true wellness isn't just possible, it's contagious."

—**Keri Glassman**, MS, RDN, CDN, Founder of Nutritious Life

"*SUPERWELL* is a beautifully structured yet deeply personal blueprint for building true vitality—rooted in powerful daily rituals, the wisdom of the 8 Pillars, and the science of personalized healing. Lauren Pronger masterfully guides you to become the architect of your own wellness journey, aligning body, mind, and spirit through intentional choices that create lasting well-being."

—**Dr. Jenelle Kim**, DACM, L.Ac., Author of *Myung Sung: The Korean Art of Living Meditation*; Founder and Formulator, JBK Wellness Labs; Taoist Longevity Expert

"I've witnessed firsthand how Lauren has lived out the SUPERWELL lifestyle—not in curated perfection, but in real, intentional, everyday choices. Her mission is proof that thriving is possible when we ground ourselves in purpose, consistency, and heart. I truly believe this message has the power to help countless others rise into their healthiest, most empowered selves."

—**Darleen Santore**, Author of *The Art of Bouncing Back: Find Your Flow to Thrive at Work and in Life — Any Time You're Off Your Game*

"As a nurse practitioner, I know firsthand how vital it is to empower my patients to take control of their health in order to live their most optimal, healthy, and fulfilling lives. Knowing Lauren personally for years, I can attest to her genuine passion for helping others achieve a truly fulfilled life. I believe *SUPERWELL* reflects that dedication. The book offers invaluable insights and practical guidance that will inspire individuals to take charge of their well-being and embark on a journey toward feeling truly great, not just good!"

—**Racquel Frisella**, MSN, APRN, AGPCNP-BC

"As the CEO of one of America's fastest growing companies, the leader of a global nonprofit, and an author, I do not have time for wellness fads or guesswork. Lauren simplifies the science so I can stay fueled, focused, and mission-ready, even on days that take me from boardrooms to national TV to children's hospitals. She makes it possible to build wellness into even the busiest schedules, bringing clarity to what truly matters for your health and teaching you how to actually follow through. Lauren is the real deal. She is certified, experienced, and genuinely walking the walk. She lives what she teaches, and it shows. Her guidance is rooted in data, facts, and lived experience, but it is her honesty, encouragement, and big heart that make it stick. She makes it possible to go after everything you care about because she helps your body keep up. And she does it without the fluff, without ego, and always with heart."

—**Erika Sinner**, CEO, Directorie; Author of *Pets Are Family*; Chief Empathy Officer, TinySuperheroes

"I have had the privilege of being in a very special friendship with Lauren for 23 years! Her dedication and commitment to her overall well-being are to be admired. *SUPERWELL* is the perfect framework that has a permanent imprint on my health and wellness!"

—**Heather Zone**, Member of the SUPERWELL Community

"The *SUPERWELL* lifestyle is a game-changer, bringing clarity, balance, and inspiration to anyone seeking lasting wellness. Watching Lauren embody and share her powerful insights has transformed the way my family approaches and prioritizes well-being and has inspired countless others, at any age, to feel empowered and in control of their health."

—**Kristin Ficery**, Member of the SUPERWELL Community

# SUPERWELL

## YOUR ULTIMATE BLUEPRINT TO WELLNESS AND WELLBEING

**LAUREN PRONGER**

# SUPERWELL™
*Your Blueprint to Wellness and Wellbeing*
Lauren Pronger

Published by Everwell Publishing, St. Louis, MO
Copyright ©2025 Lauren Pronger
All rights reserved.

No part of this publication may be reproduced, stored in a retrieval system, or transmitted in any form or by any means, electronic, mechanical, photocopying, recording, scanning, or otherwise, except as permitted under Section 107 or 108 of the 1976 United States Copyright Act, without the prior written permission of the Publisher. Requests to the Publisher for permission should be addressed to the Permissions Department, Everwell Publishing, Lauren@wellinspiredtravels.com

Limit of Liability/Disclaimer of Warranty: While the publisher and author have used their best efforts in preparing this book, they make no representations or warranties with respect to the accuracy or completeness of the contents of this book and specifically disclaim any implied warranties of merchantability or fitness for a particular purpose. No warranty may be created or extended by sales representatives or written sales materials. The advice and strategies contained herein may not be suitable for your situation. You should consult with a professional where appropriate. Neither the publisher nor the author shall be liable for any loss of profit or any other commercial damages, including but not limited to special, incidental, consequential, or other damages.

The product information and advice provided (in this book) are intended for general informational purposes only. The author and publisher of this book have made every effort to ensure that the content is accurate and up-to-date at the time of publication. However, they make no representations or warranties of any kind, express or implied, about the completeness, accuracy, reliability, suitability, or availability of the information, products, or services contained in this book for any purpose.

***The information contained in this book is meant for informational and educational purposes only and is not intended to be a substitute for the medical advice of physicians. The reader should regularly consult a physician in matters relating to his/her health and particularly with respect to dietary guidelines and the use of supplements.***

Project Management and Book Design: DavisCreativePublishing.com
Cover and Interior Design: Missy Asikainen
Editor: Kerri Landis

Library of Congress Cataloging-in-Publication Data
Names: Pronger, Lauren, author.
Title: Superwell : your ultimate blueprint to wellness and wellbeing / Lauren Pronger.
Description: St. Louis, MO : Everwell Publishing, [2025]
Identifiers: LCCN: 2025907862 | ISBN: 9798998676109 (paperback) |
     9798998676116 (ebook)
Subjects: LCSH: Well-being. | Health. | Holistic medicine. | Stress management. |
     Burn out (Psychology) | Biological rhythms. | Mind and body. | BISAC: HEALTH & FITNESS / Healthy Living. | HEALTH & FITNESS / Women's Health. | HEALTH & FITNESS / General.
Classification: LCC: RA776.9 .B53 2025 | DDC: 613--dc23

**ATTENTION CORPORATIONS, UNIVERSITIES, COLLEGES, AND PROFESSIONAL ORGANIZATIONS:**
Quantity discounts are available on bulk purchases of this book for educational, gift purposes, or as premiums for increasing magazine subscriptions or renewals. Special books or book excerpts can also be created to fit specific needs. For information, please contact Lauren Pronger, Everwell Publishing, Lauren@wellinspiredtravels.com, Laurenpronger.com

To my husband, Chris, my rock, my partner, and my greatest champion, your unwavering love, encouragement, and belief in me have been the foundation for everything I have built.

To my children, Jack, George, and Lilah, you are my heart and my inspiration. Every word in these pages is a reflection of the love I have for you and the life I hope you live: vibrant, strong, joyful, and deeply connected to what matters most.

This book is my gift to you, my legacy, a blueprint not just for wellness, but for living fully and intentionally. May it guide you, and our family for generations to come, toward a life of strength, vitality, and wholehearted wellbeing.

# CONTENTS

Introduction .................................................... 1
Striving for SUPERWELL—Together ................................ 7
Building Your Holistic Tool Belt: The Power of Personalized Healing ............. 11
Epigenetics: You Are the Captain of Your Wellness Journey .................. 15
The 8 Pillars: Building Your Blueprint for Whole-Body Wellness ............... 17
Start Here: Navigating Your SUPERWELL Blueprint ..................... 21

## A.M. HABITS

Natural Awakening ................................................ 28
Grounding Ritual ................................................. 32
SUPERWELL Morning Gut Elixir ....................................... 37
SUPERWELL Wellness Ice Cubes ...................................... 41
SUPERWELL Signature Bone Broth .................................... 44
5 SUPERWELL Gut Health Facts You Need to Know ........................ 46
Supplement Stack ................................................. 48
Start Strong: Why a Savory Breakfast Is a SUPERWELL Non-Negotiable ........ 51
How to Build the Ultimate Savory Breakfast Plate ........................ 53
SUPERWELL Breakfast Favorites ..................................... 56
Multitasking with Intention: Red Light, BioMat, & Matcha Mornings ............. 67
BioMat Brilliance: Harnessing Infrared Heat for Cellular Vitality ............... 68
Matcha Mastery: A Smarter Energy Solution for Mind & Body ................ 70
Glow Rituals as Nervous System Nourishment ........................... 76
A.M. Glass Skin Routine ............................................ 79
Contrast Therapy: Mastering the Elements ............................. 82
Sauna Sanctuary: The Science of Heat for Detox,
    Longevity, & Deep Restoration .................................... 86
Sweat, Stack, & Savor:
    Habit Stacking for the Ultimate Sauna Ritual .......................... 88
What Are the Benefits of Dry Brushing? ................................ 90
Creative Ways to Experience Heat Shock Therapy ........................ 91
Cold Shock Therapy: Mastering the Stress Switch ........................ 95

5 Powerful Reasons to Activate Your Brown Fat with Cold Shock . . . . . . . . . . . . . . 98
Creative Ways to Experience Cold Shock Therapy . . . . . . . . . . . . . . . . . . . . . . . . . . . 99
Gear Shifts to SUPERWELL . . . . . . . . . . . . . . . . . . . . . . . . . . . . . . . . . . . . . . . . . . . . . 102
Heavy Lifting: Strength Unleashed . . . . . . . . . . . . . . . . . . . . . . . . . . . . . . . . . . . . . . 104
The 20-Minute Momentum Hack:
    Trick Your Brain, Transform Your Day . . . . . . . . . . . . . . . . . . . . . . . . . . . . . . . . 106
Breaking Free from the Cardio Hamster Wheel:
    Train Smarter, Not Harder . . . . . . . . . . . . . . . . . . . . . . . . . . . . . . . . . . . . . . . . . 107
How to Train Your Heart Without Destroying Your Hormones . . . . . . . . . . . . . . . . 108
The Magic of Gentle Movement: Treat Your Body with Kindness . . . . . . . . . . . . . 109
Strength Training for Women & Longevity . . . . . . . . . . . . . . . . . . . . . . . . . . . . . . . . 110
Strength Is Your Superpower . . . . . . . . . . . . . . . . . . . . . . . . . . . . . . . . . . . . . . . . . . . 111
The Beginner's Guide to Strength Training for Women's Longevity . . . . . . . . . . . . 112
Essential Stretches for Relaxation & Flexibility . . . . . . . . . . . . . . . . . . . . . . . . . . . . 114
Basic Mat Pilates Exercises . . . . . . . . . . . . . . . . . . . . . . . . . . . . . . . . . . . . . . . . . . . . 116
10 Benefits of Pilates Movement . . . . . . . . . . . . . . . . . . . . . . . . . . . . . . . . . . . . . . . 120
Glucose Garbage Dump . . . . . . . . . . . . . . . . . . . . . . . . . . . . . . . . . . . . . . . . . . . . . . . 122
Lauren's SUPERWELL Pep Talk . . . . . . . . . . . . . . . . . . . . . . . . . . . . . . . . . . . . . . . . . 123
The SUPERWELL 12-Ingredient Protein Milkshake . . . . . . . . . . . . . . . . . . . . . . . . . 127
Why It Works: A Deeper Look at the Benefits . . . . . . . . . . . . . . . . . . . . . . . . . . . . . 128
The Importance of Clean, Filtered Water . . . . . . . . . . . . . . . . . . . . . . . . . . . . . . . . . 132
Time-Saving, Soul-Fueling Tips for A.M. Success . . . . . . . . . . . . . . . . . . . . . . . . . . 134
Take the Lead: Mastering Your Morning Momentum . . . . . . . . . . . . . . . . . . . . . . . 138
The SUPERWELL Way to 80/20 Living . . . . . . . . . . . . . . . . . . . . . . . . . . . . . . . . . . . 136
SUPERWELL On-the-Go Bento Box . . . . . . . . . . . . . . . . . . . . . . . . . . . . . . . . . . . . . 139
SUPERWELL Pro Travel Elixir Hacks . . . . . . . . . . . . . . . . . . . . . . . . . . . . . . . . . . . . . 142
SUPERWELL Greens & Glow-Ups . . . . . . . . . . . . . . . . . . . . . . . . . . . . . . . . . . . . . . . 144
SUPERWELL Soups . . . . . . . . . . . . . . . . . . . . . . . . . . . . . . . . . . . . . . . . . . . . . . . . . . 150
SUPERWELL Drizzles & Dips . . . . . . . . . . . . . . . . . . . . . . . . . . . . . . . . . . . . . . . . . . . 154

## P.M. HABIT STACKING ROUTINE

P.M. Habit Stacking: Where Evening Rhythm Meets Restorative Power . . . . . . . . 158

The SUPERWELL Glucose Flow:
Eat Smart, Stabilize Blood Sugar, Thrive Daily . . . . . . . . . . . . . . . . . . . . . . . . . . 161

Pre-Meal Strategy: Set the Stage for Success . . . . . . . . . . . . . . . . . . . . . . . . . . . . 162

The Order Matters: How to Eat Your Meal Like a SUPERWELL Superstar . . . . . . . 166

"Yes" Foods to Enjoy Closer to Bedtime . . . . . . . . . . . . . . . . . . . . . . . . . . . . . . . . 168

"No" Foods to Avoid Closer to Bedtime . . . . . . . . . . . . . . . . . . . . . . . . . . . . . . . . . 170

SUPERWELL Cheat Sheet: Understanding Macros . . . . . . . . . . . . . . . . . . . . . . . . 173

Strong > Skinny: Redefining the Why Behind What You Eat . . . . . . . . . . . . . . . . 177

SUPERWELL P.M. Plates . . . . . . . . . . . . . . . . . . . . . . . . . . . . . . . . . . . . . . . . . . . . . . 179

Evening Walk Magic: Your SUPERWELL Secret Weapon . . . . . . . . . . . . . . . . . . . 189

Digital Dimming: The Science & Soul of a Tech Detox . . . . . . . . . . . . . . . . . . . . . 192

Evening Ritual . . . . . . . . . . . . . . . . . . . . . . . . . . . . . . . . . . . . . . . . . . . . . . . . . . . . . . 194

SUPERWELL Zen Sleep Tool Kit . . . . . . . . . . . . . . . . . . . . . . . . . . . . . . . . . . . . . . . . 196

Magnesium Bath Ritual: A SUPERWELL Reset for Body & Mind . . . . . . . . . . . . . 201

Parasympathetic Power: My Evening Meditative Reset . . . . . . . . . . . . . . . . . . . . 204

My SUPERWELL Nighttime Ritual . . . . . . . . . . . . . . . . . . . . . . . . . . . . . . . . . . . . . . 206

SUPERWELL Glowing Skin PM Routine—
Retinol & Acid Slough-Off Nights . . . . . . . . . . . . . . . . . . . . . . . . . . . . . . . . . . . . 208

Smart Supplementation + Nourishment . . . . . . . . . . . . . . . . . . . . . . . . . . . . . . . . 214

Literary Escape . . . . . . . . . . . . . . . . . . . . . . . . . . . . . . . . . . . . . . . . . . . . . . . . . . . . . 218

Lights Out: Your Evening Blueprint for SUPERWELL Sleep . . . . . . . . . . . . . . . . . . 221

Conclusion: The Journey to SUPERWELL—Together . . . . . . . . . . . . . . . . . . . . . . 222

## APPENDIX

Meet Your SUPERWELL-ish Living BFF . . . . . . . . . . . . . . . . . . . . . . . . . . . . . . . . . . 227

SUPERWELL Mantras . . . . . . . . . . . . . . . . . . . . . . . . . . . . . . . . . . . . . . . . . . . . . . . . 230

Your SUPERWELL Alignment Check-Ins . . . . . . . . . . . . . . . . . . . . . . . . . . . . . . . . . 233

SUPERWELL Sunday Setup . . . . . . . . . . . . . . . . . . . . . . . . . . . . . . . . . . . . . . . . . . . 236

SUPERWELL Meditation Mantras . . . . . . . . . . . . . . . . . . . . . . . . . . . . . . . . . . . . . . 238

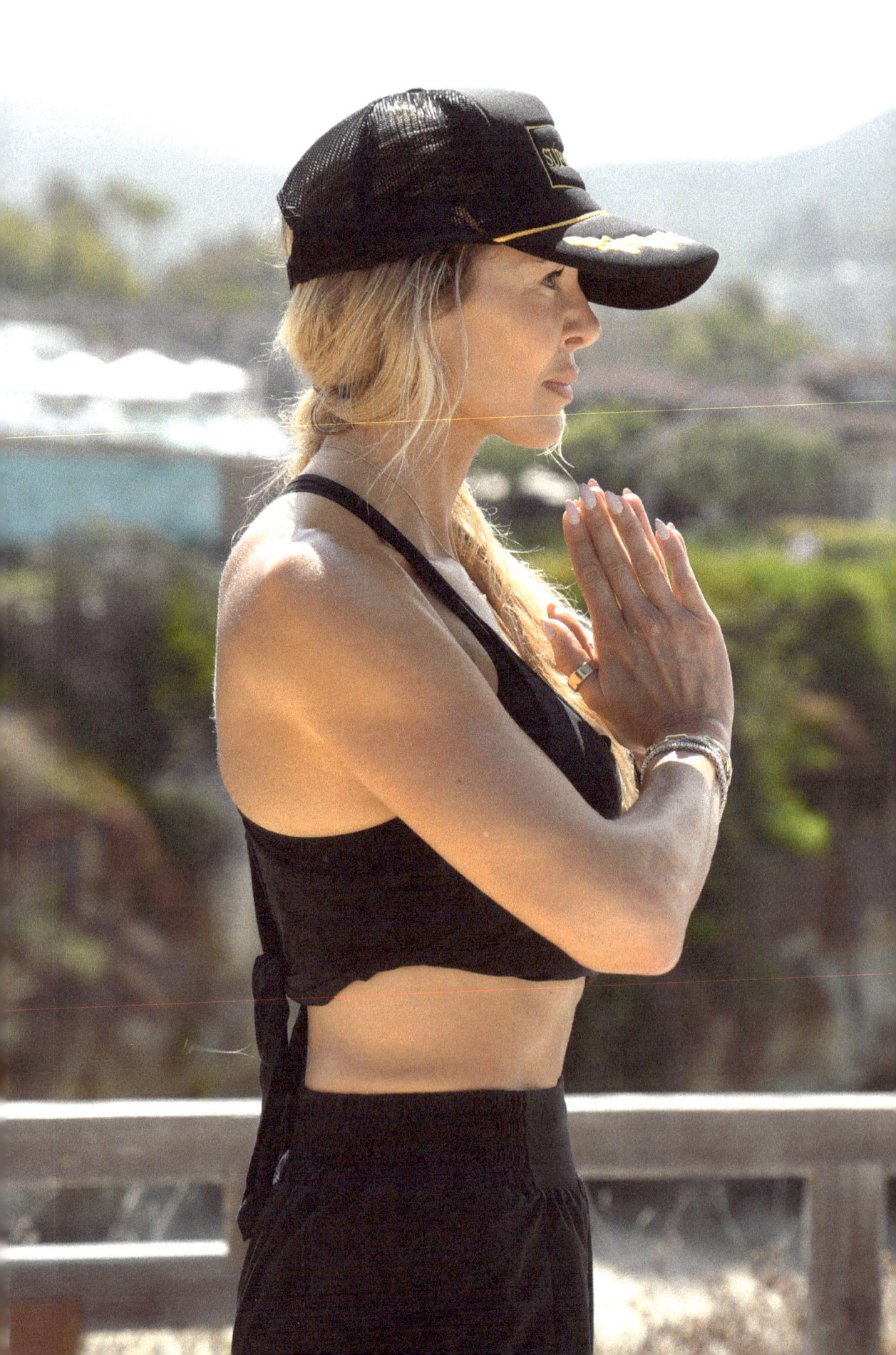

## INTRODUCTION:

# I AM THE WELL— STRIVING TO BE SUPERWELL

Every morning, before my feet even touch the ground, I remind myself of one simple truth: I am the well, striving to be SUPERWELL. Emphasis on *striving*. Because I am not perfect, and I don't pretend to be. I don't have all the answers, but what I do have is the unwavering belief that every single day, I have the power to make choices that support my body, mind, and spirit. And I am here to guide you in doing the same.

This book isn't about selling you a quick fix. It's not a diet, a supplement, or a magic workout plan. It's about something much bigger. It's about following a blueprint for living with intention, vitality, and resilience. It's about reclaiming control in a world that constantly pulls us toward stress, distraction, and burnout.

Inside these pages, you will find a structured, yet flexible, blueprint designed to help you become the driver of your own health. To step boldly into the captain's seat of your wellbeing. To make the conscious decision, day after day, to strive toward the strongest, calmest, most grounded version of yourself. Not through extremes, but through daily alignment, deliberate action, and the power of showing up for your life on purpose.

## THE ROOTS OF MY JOURNEY

My passion for health and wellness wasn't something I stumbled upon; it's something that's lived in me since I was a little girl. From a young age, I was deeply curious about how the body works, how we heal, and what it truly takes to live a vibrant, energized life from the inside out. When I was growing up, my family, like many families, faced its fair share of health challenges; instead of feeling helpless, I felt called. I found myself constantly asking questions, watching closely, and gravitating toward anything that offered insight into feeling better, living longer, and glowing from within. That early spark, equal parts wonder and determination, planted the seed for what would eventually become the SUPERWELL Living Method. But it wouldn't be until years later, during my own personal health reckoning, that I would learn just how powerful those instincts really were.

As I grew older, life continued to test me in ways I never expected. In the fall of 2011, everything seemed to come crashing down at once. My husband, Chris, who was one of the top NHL defensemen, suffered a career-ending concussion that left him bedridden. I couldn't leave his side. At the same time, my father suffered a stroke, and my mother was diagnosed with breast cancer for the first time. I was stretched beyond my limits emotionally, physically, and mentally. I had three young children depending on me, yet I felt like I had nothing left to give. I was completely burned out and running on fumes.

And that was the moment I knew something had to change.

## REBUILDING FROM BURNOUT ONE HABIT AT A TIME

I didn't wake up one morning with all the answers. There was no magic moment of clarity. Instead, I started habit by habit, brick by brick, rebuilding my wellbeing from the ground up. I became obsessed with understanding the human body, the nervous system, and how to truly optimize health from the inside out.

I dove deep into education, earning certifications in holistic nutrition, gut-brain health, and hormone health, as well as becoming a board-certified holistic practitioner. I graduated from the Institute for Integrative Nutrition (IIN) program and continued with three additional years of education with IIN, further deepening my knowledge.

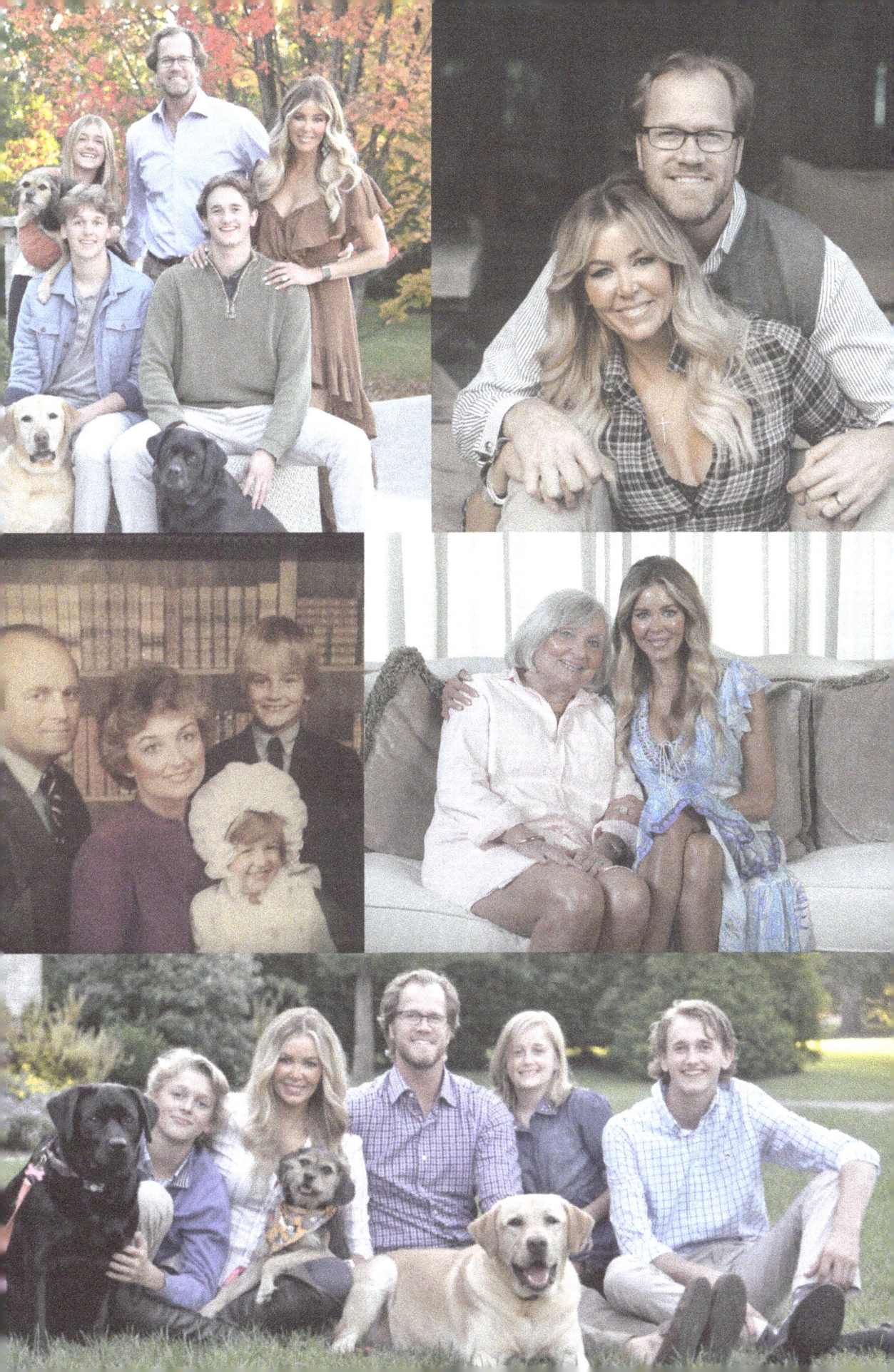

I also was certified as a master nutrition and wellness coach through the Nutritious Life Studio. I later trained as a contrast therapy guide, a breathwork instructor, and a meditation guide. I studied and became certified in two disciplines of Pilates for strength and balance.

Because here's the truth: Our society is more stressed, more inflamed, and more disconnected than ever before. We live in a world that constantly triggers our sympathetic nervous system, and the fight-or-flight response keeps us in a state of chronic stress. We are bombarded with distractions, toxins, and pressures that pull us further away from what we need most: simplicity, balance, and true wellbeing.

**But here's the good news: We have the power to take it back.**

**The SUPERWELL Living Method isn't about restriction or perfection.** It's not about chasing the latest diet trend or stocking your pantry with every new supplement. It's a return to what truly works, the foundational blueprint your body has always been asking for: a blueprint rooted in simplicity, rhythm, and trust.

This method guides you to reconnect with what matters most: how to nourish your body with real, whole foods; how to calm and regulate your nervous system; how to move with intention and honor your body's cues; and how to live with clarity, alignment, and purpose.

And the best part? This blueprint isn't something you have to buy. It already lives within you. This book simply helps you remember how to access it.

We eat our food, we soak in the morning sunlight, we breathe in fresh air, we move our bodies, we train our minds, and we nurture our relationships—all of which have the power to radically transform our health when done with intention.

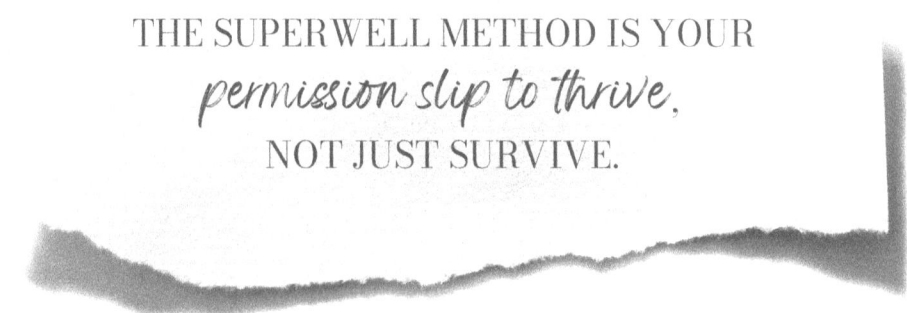

THE SUPERWELL METHOD IS YOUR *permission slip to thrive,* NOT JUST SURVIVE.

## WHY THIS BOOK? WHY NOW?

I wrote this book because I believe the world needs it now more than ever. We need a new definition of health: one that isn't about extremes, deprivation, or quick fixes. One that is about sustainability, balance, and lifelong vitality.

I want to show my children that, while genetics may play a role in our health, we are not powerless. Epigenetics teaches us that our genes are not our destiny. In fact, our lifestyle, environment, and daily habits have the power to influence which genes are activated and how they express themselves. Yes, I carry the genetic markers for heart disease, diabetes, and cancer, but does that mean I'm going to sit back and accept that fate? Absolutely not. I wake up every day with the intention to live my most optimal, SUPERWELL life—because why the heck not? If I have the choice to feel amazing, energized, and strong, I am going to take it.

And I want the same for you.

This book is my way of saying: You are in control. You are the well, and *you* hold the blueprint. Your health, your energy, your joy . . . it all starts with you. My role is simply to guide you, to cheer you on, and to equip you with the tools to build a life that feels vibrant, empowered, and deeply fulfilling.

So, let's do this together. Let's anchor into a blueprint that builds resilience. Let's create habits that support longevity, vitality, and joy. Let's wake up each day with the clarity and confidence that we have the power to shape our health and our future.

You are the well. Strive to be SUPERWELL— every single day.

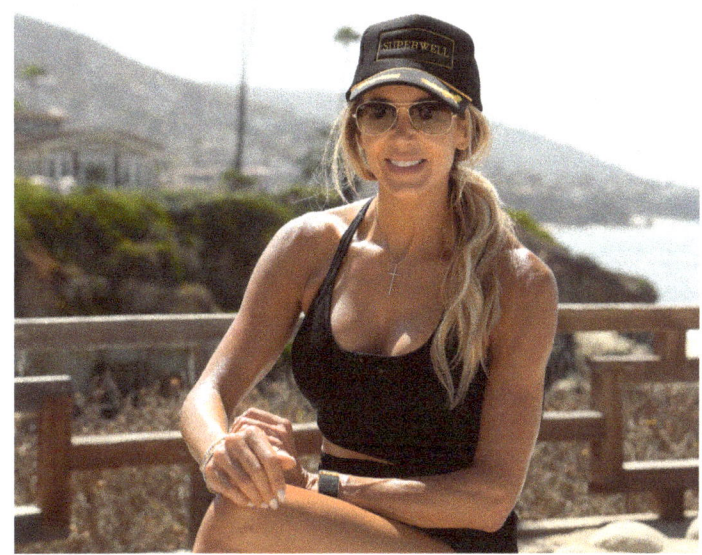

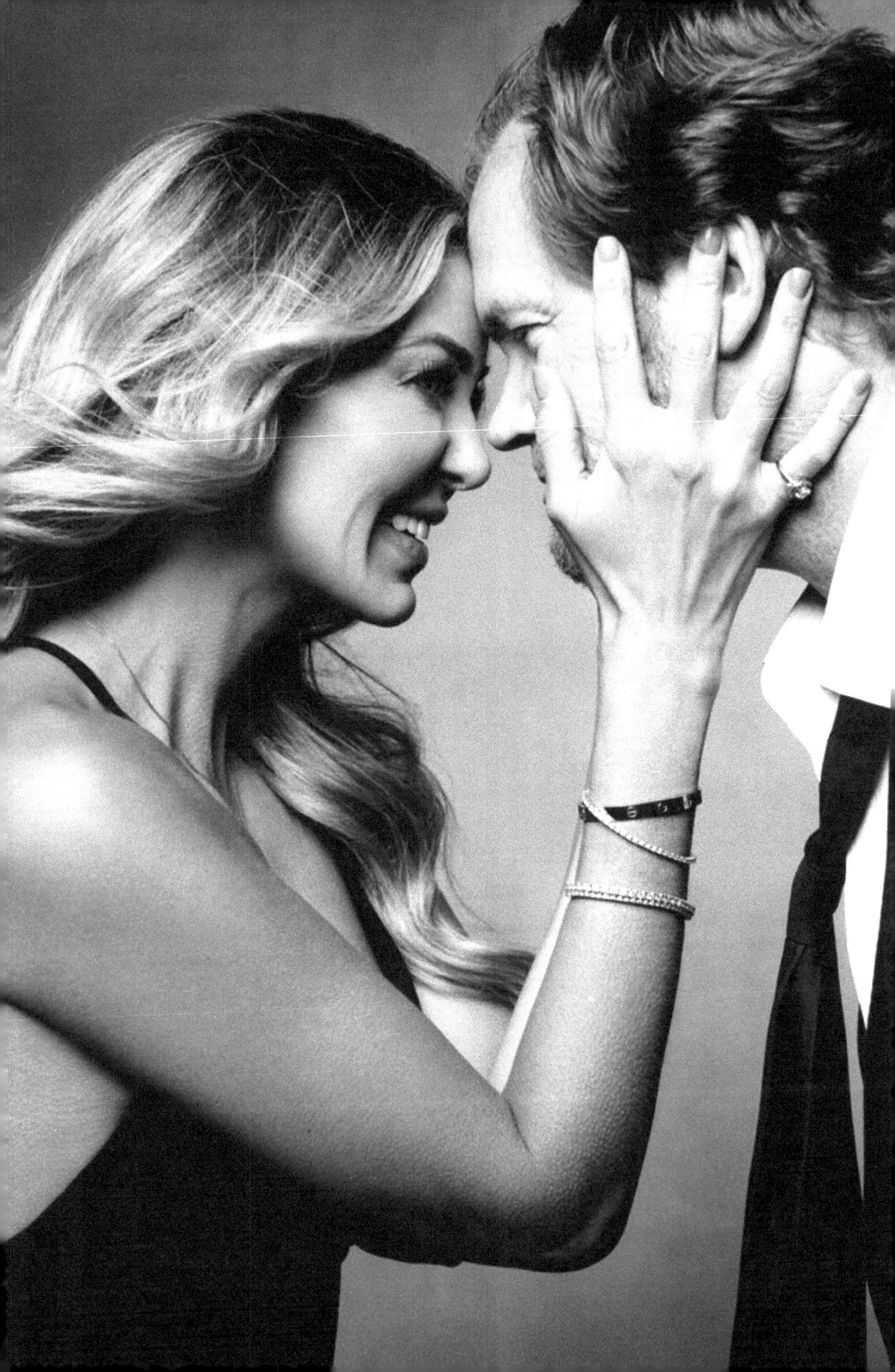

## CHRIS & LAUREN:
# STRIVING FOR SUPERWELL— TOGETHER

For 20 years, Chris played at the highest level of professional hockey, achieving what most athletes only dream of: a Stanley Cup, an Olympic gold medal, multiple All-Star selections, and induction into the Hockey Hall of Fame. But behind the accolades, behind the moments of triumph on the ice, was a life that was anything but easy . . . 16 surgeries, multiple concussions, constant physical pain, and mental battles that didn't end when the final whistle blew.

Our journey together, both as a couple and as individuals, has been a testament to resilience, adaptation, and, ultimately, transformation. The world of professional athletics is filled with incredible blessings, but it also comes with intense pressures that test every part of you . . . physically, mentally, and emotionally. We have experienced firsthand the toll that high-performance living takes on both the athlete and the family behind them. Time away from home; overnight trades; uncertainty; moves; kids switching schools; injuries that never fully heal; and the identity crisis that comes when the game no longer defines you.

Chris did not get to leave the sport on his own terms. A career-ending concussion forced an abrupt and painful transition. The identity he had built for decades—Chris Pronger, NHL defenseman, warrior on the ice—was suddenly gone. And for a long time, that loss was heavier than any trophy he had ever lifted. It was a battle that was fought in silence, in the stillness of nights where sleep wouldn't come, in the frustration of a body that wouldn't recover like it used to, and in the struggle of finding purpose beyond the rink.

As his wife, I was there through it all. I watched him fight for his health, for his mental clarity, and for a sense of self outside of the sport that had defined him. And through that struggle, something powerful happened . . . we rebuilt. Not just Chris, but both of us, together. We redesigned our lives with intention, creating something that wasn't just about surviving the aftermath of a career, but about thriving in the next chapter.

## A NEW DEFINITION OF STRENGTH

For men, strength is often tied to performance, productivity, and endurance. Whether it's in professional sports, business, or daily life, there is an unspoken expectation to push through, ignore the pain, and handle things alone. But what we have learned is that true strength comes not from ignoring what your body and mind are telling you, but from listening, adapting, and taking ownership of your health.

Chris is now in his prime years, and through the SUPERWELL Living Method, he is in the same weight, shape, and strength as he was when he won the Stanley Cup and Olympic gold medal. This is not by accident. It is the result of being intentional . . . prioritizing sleep, optimizing recovery, fueling his body with the right nutrients, and embracing breathwork, contrast therapy, and strength training as non-negotiables.

For years, he played through pain. Now, he plays for longevity. He plays for life.

## FROM THE ICE TO THE BOARDROOM: THE SUPERWELL ADVANTAGE

What we have built together through SUPERWELL Living is not just for elite athletes or those coming out of high-performance careers. This is a lifestyle that applies to anyone looking to maximize their potential, whether in business, leadership, or daily life.

The same principles that lead to success in professional sports—discipline, consistency, mindset, and recovery—are the same ones that create high-performing teams in corporate settings. Whether you are an executive, an entrepreneur, or a team leader, your ability to show up with clarity, focus, and energy directly impacts your performance, your relationships, and your overall success.

This is why we are expanding this mission beyond just personal health. We are bringing SUPERWELL into corporate wellness, team coaching, and leadership development. When individuals operate at their best, teams thrive, businesses succeed, and cultures transform.

## BUILDING A LEGACY OF HEALTH—TOGETHER

One of the biggest transformations in our journey has been learning how to support each other in the pursuit of health. For so long, we were both running in survival mode, pushing through stress, exhaustion, and burnout. Now, we prioritize our wellbeing as a couple, knowing that the stronger we are individually, the stronger we are together.

This book was written with that in mind—to inspire both men and women to take ownership of their health, to support one another in the process, and to build a life of strength, longevity, and fulfillment.

It doesn't matter if you're an athlete, a CEO, a busy parent, or someone who simply wants to feel better—the SUPERWELL Living Method offers a blueprint to help you optimize your life from the inside out.

So, the question we leave you with is this: Why settle for just "well" when you can be SUPERWELL?

It's time to take control. It's time to thrive. Let's do it together.

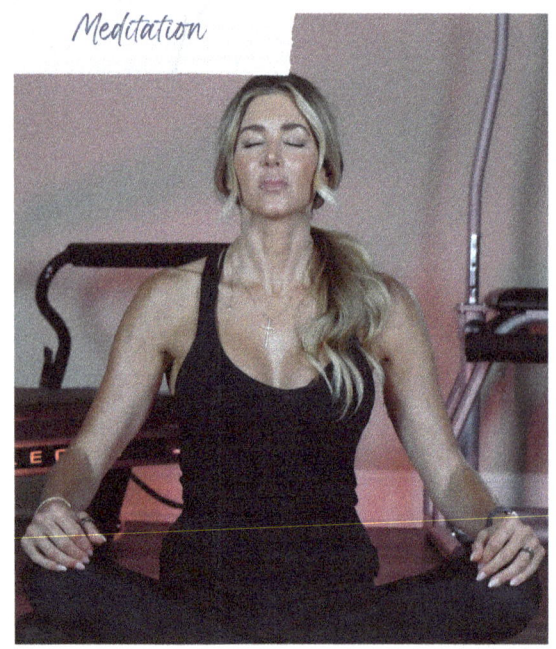
*Meditation*

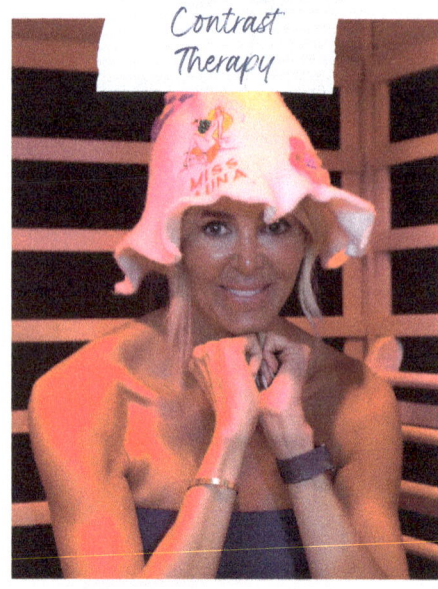
*Contrast Therapy*

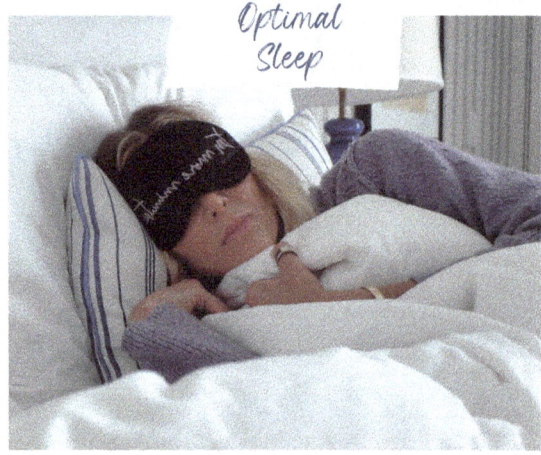
*Optimal Sleep*

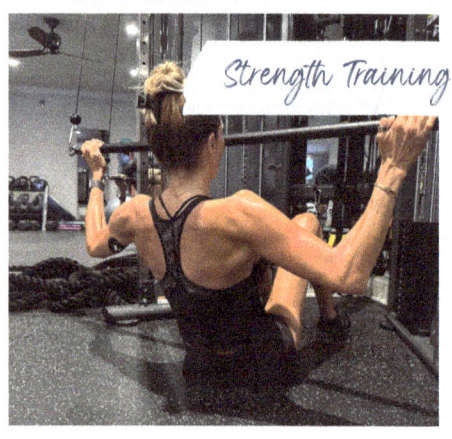
*Strength Training*

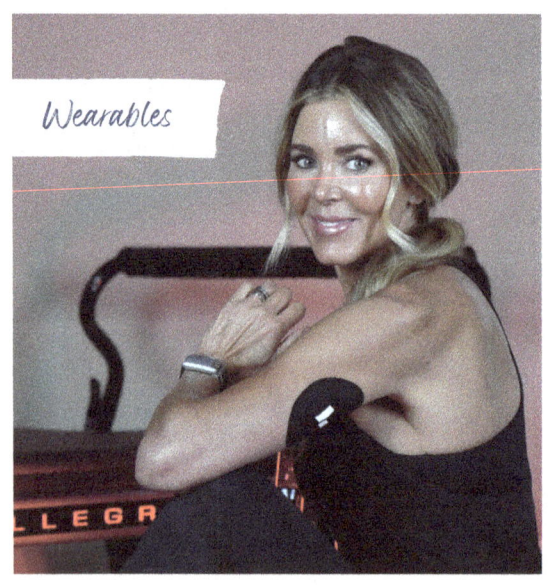
*Wearables*

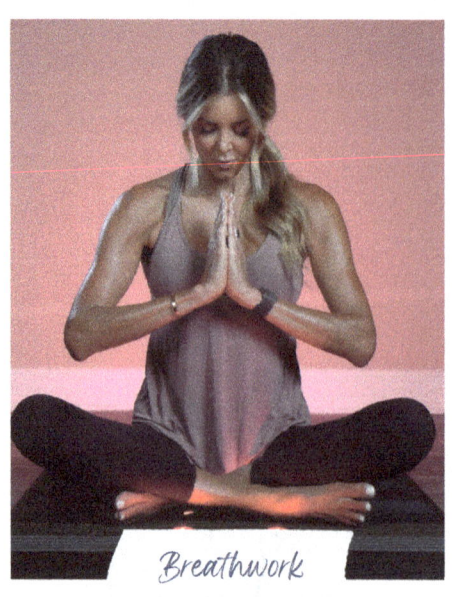
*Breathwork*

## BUILDING YOUR HOLISTIC TOOL BELT:
# THE POWER OF PERSONALIZED HEALING

Back in 2011, when I hit burnout, I felt like my body was betraying me—I was exhausted, anxious, inflamed, and completely drained. No amount of coffee could keep me going, no workout felt restorative, and sleep never seemed to be enough. I had been living in a constant state of fight-or-flight, and my body was screaming for help. That was the turning point. I knew something had to change.

Instead of looking for a quick fix, I started to build my own holistic tool belt: a collection of powerful, science-backed wellness tools that I could turn to at any moment to restore balance, calm my nervous system, and reclaim my energy. And now, I want to help you do the same.

Your holistic tool belt is unique to you. It's a set of practices, therapies, and habits that bring you back to homeostasis—your natural state of balance and vitality. Some tools bring energy; some calm the nervous system; and others optimize longevity and resilience. The key is knowing which ones to use and when.

## ESSENTIAL TOOLS FOR YOUR HOLISTIC TOOL BELT

**Meditation & Breathwork** – Whether it's meditation, guided visualization, or simple breathwork techniques like 4-7-8 breathing, these tools help shift your body into parasympathetic mode, reducing stress and promoting deep relaxation.

**Contrast Therapy** – Harnessing the power of heat and cold shock therapy (saunas + cold plunges) stimulates circulation, reduces inflammation, and builds resilience. This practice trains your nervous system to handle stress better while supporting muscle recovery and metabolic health.

**Strength Training & Lifting Heavy** – One of the most underrated longevity tools, strength training improves hormonal balance, boosts metabolism, strengthens bones, and enhances cognitive function. Your muscle is your metabolic currency . . . the more you have, the more resilient you become.

**Optimal Sleep Practices** – Sleep isn't just about rest; it's when your body heals, hormones regulate, and brain detoxification happens. Mastering circadian rhythm hacks like morning sunlight exposure, blue light blocking, and an optimized sleep routine will change your energy, mood, and longevity.

**Wearables & Bio-Tracking** – Understanding your own bio-individual body is the key to knowing what truly works for you. High-level tools like heart rate variability (HRV) tracking, continuous glucose monitors (CGMs), and sleep trackers give real-time feedback so you can adjust habits accordingly.

**Nervous System Regulation** – In our chaotic world, knowing how to shift out of stress mode is life-changing. Tools like red light therapy, acupressure mats, grounding, and vagus nerve stimulation help regulate the nervous system and restore balance when life feels overwhelming.

## WHY YOUR HOLISTIC TOOL BELT MATTERS

Life will always throw stress, uncertainty, and challenges our way. But when you have the right tools, you are equipped to handle it all with resilience.

Your holistic tool belt isn't just about wellness hacks; it's a deeply personal, intuitive collection of healing methods that help you:

- ✔ Stay grounded in times of stress
- ✔ Restore energy when burnout creeps in
- ✔ Recover faster from illness, workouts, or overwhelm
- ✔ Strengthen your body, mind, and spirit every single day

The beauty of this tool belt is that you don't need to use every tool every day, but when you know what works for your body, you will always have exactly what you need at your fingertips.

This book is here to help you build your own holistic tool belt, guided by a blueprint that honors your unique life, rhythms, and needs. When you have the right tools and a clear map for using them, you don't just survive . . . you thrive.

*SUPERWELL LIVING ISN'T ABOUT DOING MORE — it's about doing what matters.*

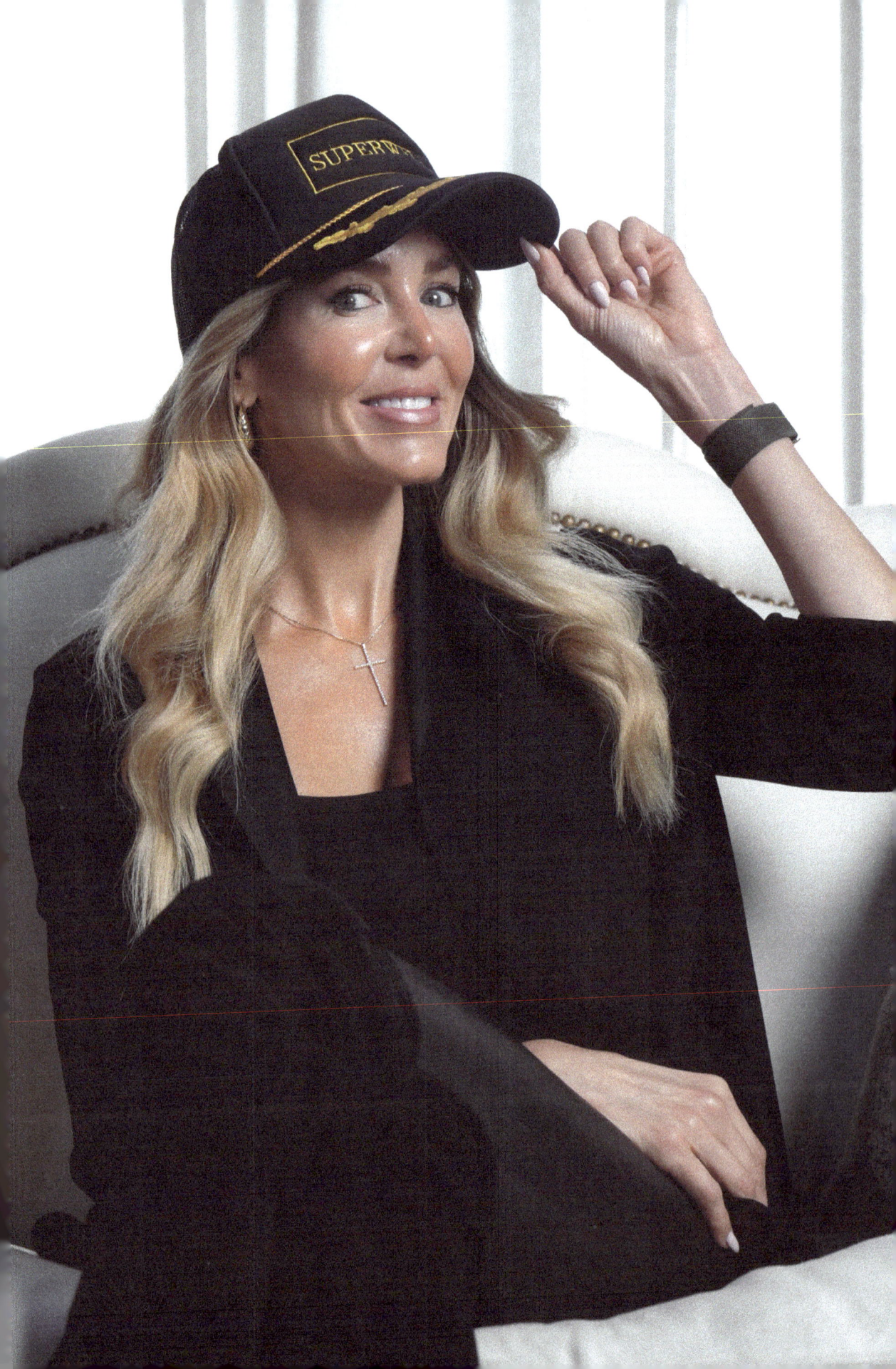

## EPIGENETICS:
# YOU ARE THE CAPTAIN OF YOUR WELLNESS JOURNEY

For as long as I can remember, I have been aware of my family health history—colon cancer, breast cancer, heart disease, and diabetes are written in my genetic code. But here's what I refuse to accept: that my genetics are my fate.

Science tells us that while we inherit our genes, we control how they express themselves. This is epigenetics—the study of how lifestyle choices influence gene activation. Think of your genes as a loaded gun, but your daily habits determine whether or not the trigger gets pulled. Every meal, movement, moment of stress, and night of sleep either supports health or pushes you toward disease.

### STEERING THE SHIP:
### YOUR DAILY HABITS = GENETIC INSURANCE

This is why I created and wear my SUPERWELL captain's hat—a symbolic hat with gold captain's wings and the SUPERWELL logo. It's a daily reminder that I am in control of my health and longevity. I refuse to let my genetic history define my future, and neither should you. Are you in the driver's seat of your health, or are you letting your genetics take the wheel?

**You Are the Captain of Your Own Wellness Journey** – Every decision you make is a course correction. You can drift aimlessly or take control, navigate with intention, and chart a path toward health, vitality, and longevity. The SUPERWELL hat is a reminder that you are in charge.

**The Captain Sign = Leadership in Your Own Life** – Captains don't drift with the current—they lead with strategy, wisdom, and action. Your health isn't something to "go with the flow" on—it requires commitment and direction. Step into the role of leader over your body, mind, and spirit.

**Time to Get in the Front Seat, Buckle Up, & Steer Your Ship** – Your choices today impact your future. Are you fueling your body with nutrient-dense foods? Moving with purpose? Prioritizing recovery? Or are you letting your wellness drift? The wheel is in your hands every single day.

**Every Small Decision Adds Up** – What you eat, how you sleep, and how you manage stress, movement, and recovery are the building blocks of your longevity. These daily choices dictate whether you thrive or merely survive. No one else can make these decisions for you—it's all in your hands.

**Be the Captain, Not the Passenger** – The world is filled with distractions, quick-fix fads, and noise telling you to sit back and coast. But optimal health isn't passive—it's intentional. Take the lead, set your course, and don't wait for permission to go all in on your wellbeing.

**Your Health Isn't a Predetermined Fate, It's a Lifelong Journey That You Get to Navigate** – You are not powerless against your genetics. Every choice you make is a stroke of the pen rewriting your family health history. The question is, are you ready to take the wheel and lead yourself toward a future of strength, vitality, and longevity?

## THE 8 PILLARS:

# BUILDING YOUR BLUEPRINT FOR WHOLE-BODY WELLNESS

Before diving into the daily habit stacks that form the heart of this book, it's essential to understand the foundation they rest upon: the 8 Pillars of SUPERWELL Living. These pillars are more than wellness buzzwords; they are the core framework behind your *ultimate blueprint to wellness and wellbeing*. Each pillar represents a vital dimension of holistic health, and together, they form a system of balance, clarity, and optimization. You will find these themes intentionally woven throughout the A.M.-to-P.M. rituals in this book because to live SUPERWELL is to live in rhythm with your body, your environment, and your highest self. Whether it's through the lens of nourishing nutrition, emotional wellness, restorative sleep, or biorhythmic alignment, each pillar supports and reinforces the others, creating an integrated map for sustainable vitality. As you move through the daily practices, you will begin to see how the 8 Pillars interconnect and how building your own blueprint starts with understanding them.

## 8 PILLARS TO SUPERWELL LIVING

### 1. WELL-AGING
Harness the secrets of longevity and vitality, blending cutting-edge science with holistic practices to promote a vibrant, youthful life. This pillar focuses on maintaining strength, energy, and resilience throughout all stages of life.

### 2. OPTIMAL SLEEP
Prioritize restorative sleep as the foundation of optimal health, ensuring deep, energizing rest that rejuvenates the body and mind. This pillar supports the development of consistent sleep patterns to enhance recovery and overall wellbeing.

### 3. BALANCED FLOW
Achieve physical harmony and resilience through dynamic movement and intentional practices that balance the body's energy. This pillar promotes fluidity and strength, ensuring a well-balanced and agile physique.

### 4. EMOTIONAL WELLNESS
Cultivate inner peace and emotional resilience by nurturing your mental and emotional wellbeing. This pillar emphasizes the importance of mindfulness, emotional intelligence, and stress management for a balanced life, encouraging you to live mostly in the parasympathetic nervous system state.

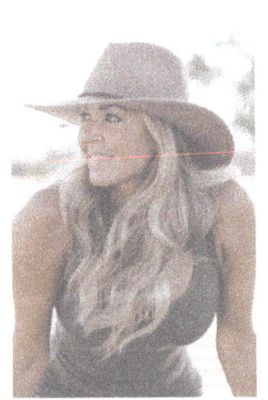
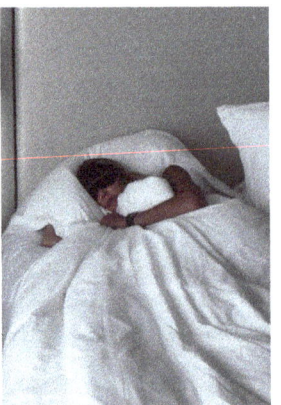
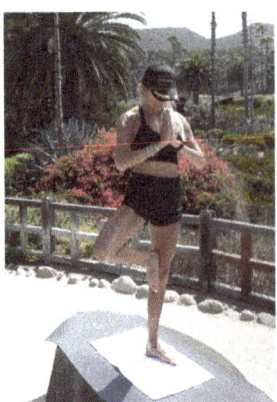
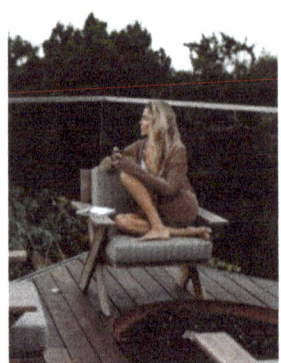

5. **NATURE CONNECTION**

   Reconnect with the natural world to restore balance and enhance your overall wellness. This pillar leverages the healing power of nature, encouraging immersion in natural environments to rejuvenate the mind, body, and spirit.

6. **NOURISHING NUTRITION**

   Fuel your body with colorful, vibrant, nutrient-dense foods that power energy, cellular repair, and sustained radiance. This pillar highlights the importance of personalized nutrition to support metabolic health, hormonal balance, and long-term strength—nourishing not just your body, but the full-spectrum life you are meant to live.

7. **BIORHYTHM/MINDFULNESS**

   Align your life with your body's natural rhythms through mindful practices that enhance clarity, focus, and emotional balance. This pillar supports the synchronization of daily habits with your internal cycles, fostering both mental and physical harmony.

8. **SOULFUL CONNECTION**

   Deepen your connection to your higher self and the world around you, fostering a life of purpose and simplicity. This pillar encourages spiritual growth and a return to the basics, focusing on what truly matters in life.

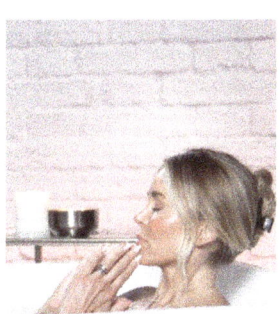 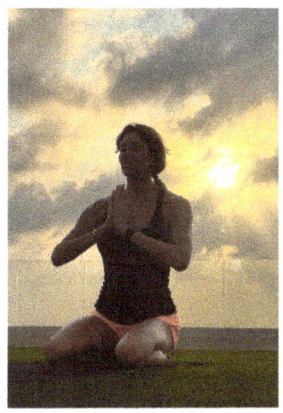 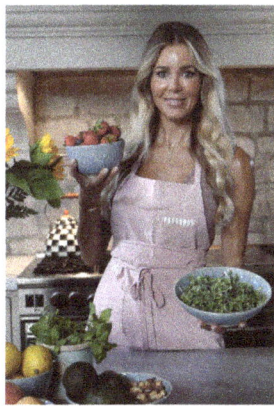 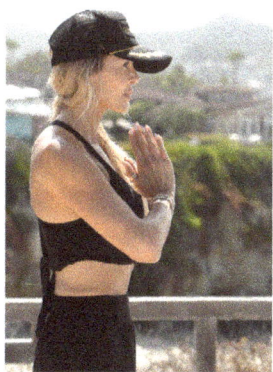

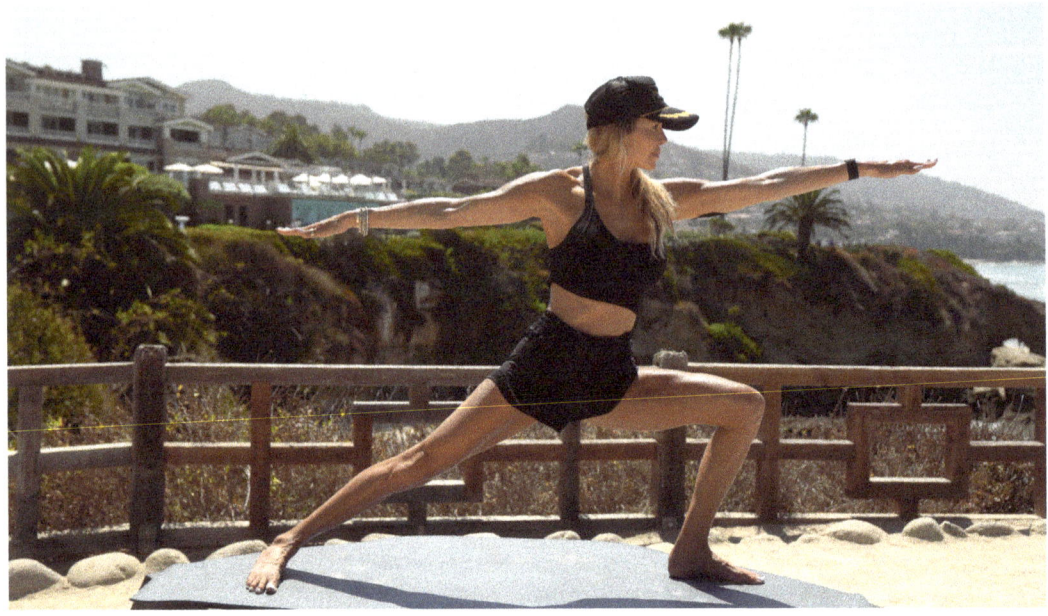

## WHY THE NUMBER 8 IS SACRED TO MY SUPERWELL LIVING METHOD

The number 8 holds profound significance in my life and serves as the foundation of the SUPERWELL Living Method. It embodies balance, continuity, and the boundless potential that life offers. Much like the infinity symbol it resembles, the number 8 represents the continuous flow and interconnectedness of all aspects of health and wellness. This idea of cyclical harmony is integral to the SUPERWELL Living Method, where every element is connected, creating a life of vitality and fulfillment. The 8 Pillars within this method are not just concepts, but a lifestyle, each one representing a crucial facet of balanced living. By embracing these 8 Pillars, you are not merely striving for balance; you are living it, with the number 8 guiding you toward a harmonious existence where wellness is not only achieved but also sustained in every aspect of life.

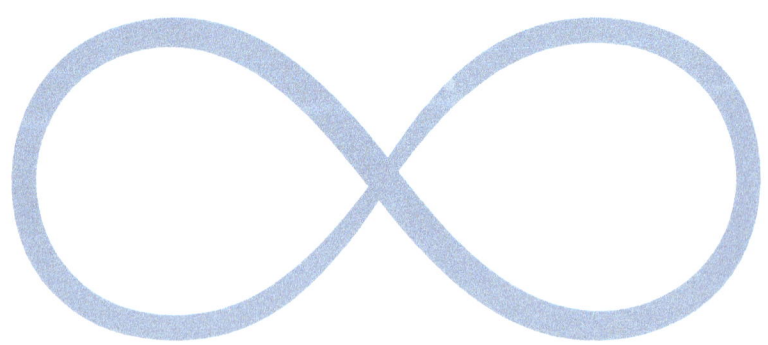

## START HERE:

# NAVIGATING YOUR SUPERWELL BLUEPRINT

*No Perfection Required, Just Progress*

### WELLNESS SHOULDN'T BE THIS OVERWHELMING

If you have ever felt exhausted from trying to keep up with all the wellness noise, you are not alone. Every day, there is a new supplement, a new diet trend, a new "must-do" routine promising to be *the answer* to better health. It's exhausting. And honestly? It's not working.

Women today are more burned out than ever before. We are juggling careers, families, responsibilities, and endless to-do lists, often putting our own wellbeing on the back burner. We try to keep up with the latest wellness advice, but instead of feeling better, we feel more overwhelmed, more drained, and more confused about what actually works.

I know this because I have been there. I have been through total burnout—physically, emotionally, and mentally. I have tried all the things, only to realize that true, sustainable wellness isn't about adding more—it's about simplifying.

That's why I created SUPERWELL Living.

This book is your blueprint to cut through the clutter and reset your health with foundational habits that actually last. No gimmicks. No impossible routines. Just a clear, simple method designed to help you feel your best every single day.

## WHAT YOU WILL FIND IN THIS BOOK

- ✔ Ditch the confusion and learn what actually works for you—not what's trending.
- ✔ Reset your health with foundational habits that fit into your busy life.
- ✔ Overcome burnout by tapping into the habits of high performers who stay energized.
- ✔ Achieve next-level health with real, science-backed strategies for optimal living.
- ✔ Turn daily routines into powerful wellness rituals that restore and strengthen you.

I created this book as a solution to the overwhelm. It's not another wellness trend; it's a blueprint back to balance, energy, and clarity.

## THINK OF THIS AS YOUR BURNOUT INSURANCE

We are living in survival mode. Stress and exhaustion have become *normal,* but that doesn't mean they have to be *your* normal.

Your body is designed to heal, to recharge, to be strong—but only if you give it what it needs. The problem isn't that you are not *doing enough*—it's that you have been told the wrong things. You have been sold quick fixes instead of real, lasting solutions.

The SUPERWELL Living Method is different. It's about going back to what actually works. It's about building habits that protect your energy, restore your resilience, and bring you back to feeling like *you* again.

Think of this book as your burnout insurance—your guide to feeling stronger, calmer, and more energized, without adding more stress to your plate.

## CUTTING THROUGH THE NOISE—BACK TO BASICS

Let's be honest: Wellness has become overly complicated. Everywhere you turn, someone is selling a new diet, a new program, a new magic pill. But real wellness? It's been the same for centuries.

If we look at how our grandparents and great-grandparents lived, they weren't doing extreme workouts, tracking every macro, or biohacking their way through life. They focused on simple, effective habits that worked—eating whole foods, moving daily, getting sunlight, prioritizing rest, and nurturing community.

That's what this book is about: Getting back to the core of what truly makes us feel well.

- ✘ No more trying to keep up with every new wellness trend.
- ✘ No more overcomplicating health with impossible routines.
- ✘ No more burning out in the name of "self-care."

Instead, you will learn how to:

- ✔ Simplify your approach to wellness so it fits into your life, not the other way around.
- ✔ Build habits that last—without the stress or frustration.
- ✔ Reclaim your energy, resilience, and vitality with small, consistent shifts.

Because wellness doesn't have to be hard—it just has to be sustainable.

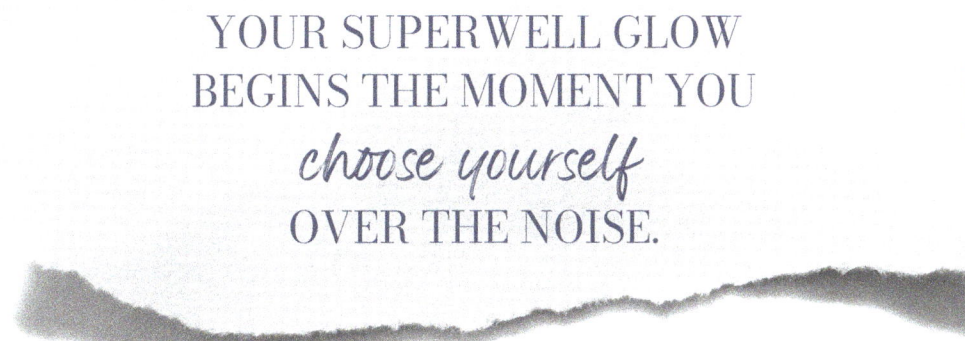

YOUR SUPERWELL GLOW BEGINS THE MOMENT YOU *choose yourself* OVER THE NOISE.

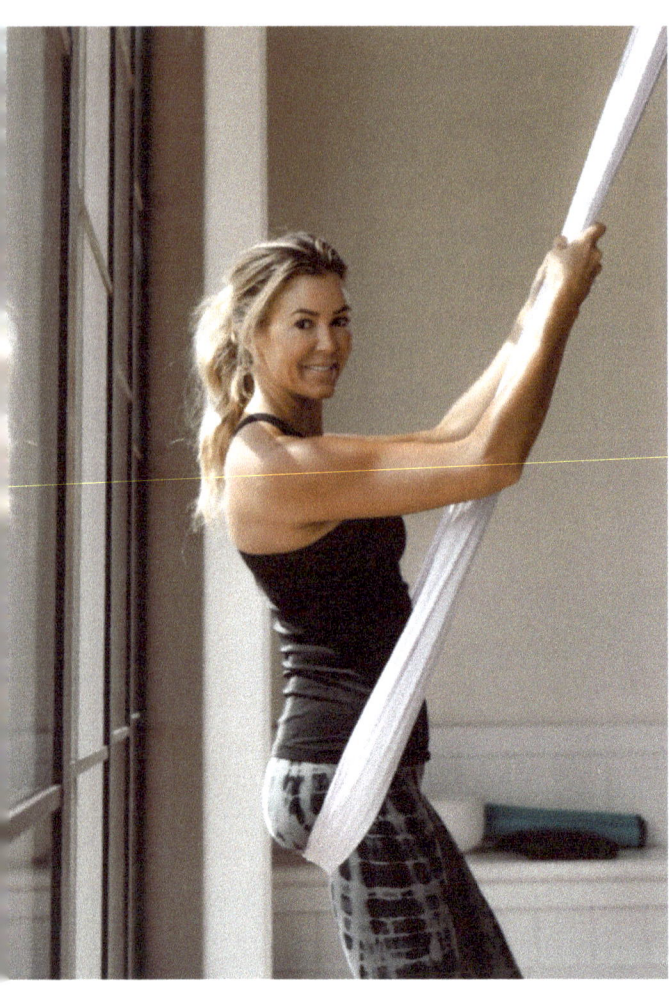

## WHY SETTLE FOR "WELL" WHEN YOU CAN BE SUPERWELL?

You deserve more than just getting by. You deserve to wake up energized, strong, and at peace in your own skin.

That's the vision behind SUPERWELL Living. This book is your invitation to step away from the noise, the overwhelm, and the exhaustion, and step into a way of living that is simple, sustainable, and truly transformative.

By the time you finish reading this book, you will have a clear, doable blueprint to feeling not just well—but SUPERWELL.

## HOW TO USE THIS BLUEPRINT

Let me start by saying this clearly: You are not expected to practice every habit in this book every single day. I don't even do that—and I created this method.

The SUPERWELL Living Method was never designed to overwhelm you, stress you out, or push you into perfectionism. That would go completely against the whole point of living SUPERWELL, because true wellbeing isn't found in hustle. It's found in flow, grace, and alignment with what your mind, body, and spirit need right now.

This book is your *blueprint, a flexible,* adaptable guide to help you build your own wellness rhythm based on the season of life you are in. Some weeks, your nervous system might be crying out for rest and regulation. Other times, your body might need movement, strength, and circulation. And maybe you are just here because your sleep is off, your digestion is sluggish, or your energy has flatlined. No matter where you are starting, you are in the right place.

So, how should you use this book?

Start by scanning the table of contents and asking yourself: *What area of my life feels the most out of sync?*

- ✔ If it's sleep, flip to the evening rituals and recovery tools.
- ✔ If it's stress, start with nervous system regulation and breathwork.
- ✔ If it's low energy or mood, look at blood sugar support, movement, or grounding practices.
- ✔ If you are feeling stagnant, the movement and flow chapter may be your best place to begin.

Each section is packed with habits, tools, and knowledge that I personally return to again and again. But I didn't build this knowledge overnight, and I don't expect you to either. Instead, treat this as a *choose-your-own-adventure guide.* Try one or two habits per week. See how they feel in your body and in your life. Add what works. Release what doesn't. Let each success build your momentum, and soon you will have your own personalized rhythm—your own *blueprint*—for living SUPERWELL.

And remember, this is a lifelong method. One that supports real people with real lives, responsibilities, and imperfections. You will revisit different pillars at different times, and that's the beauty of it.

So take a breath, let go of pressure, and allow this book to be the compassionate guide it was meant to be. You are not behind. You are simply building—habit by habit, choice by choice—the strongest, calmest, most aligned version of yourself.

Let's begin.

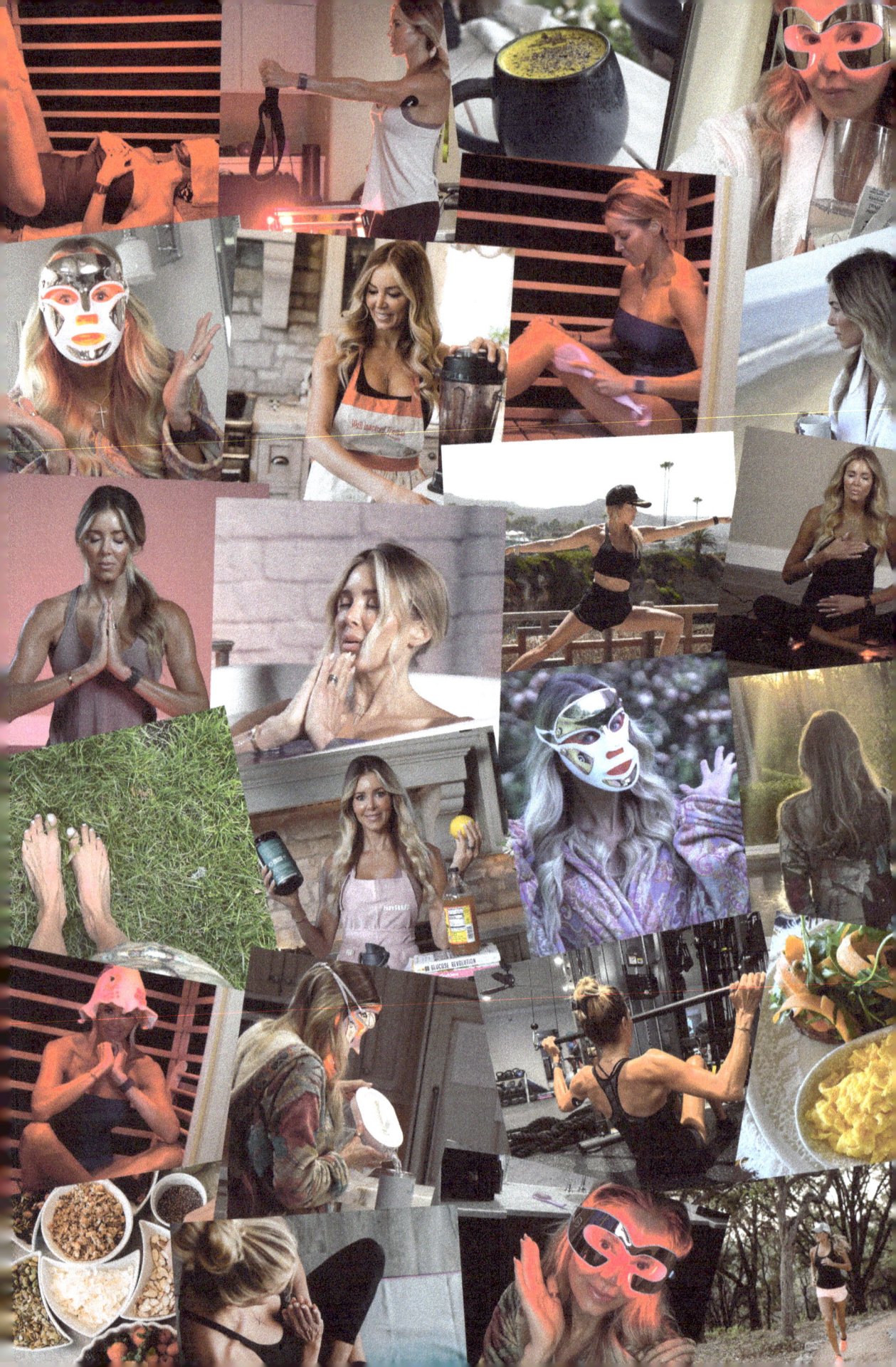

# A.M.
# HABITS

SUPERWELL

# NATURAL AWAKENING

The way you wake up sets the tone for your entire day and your long-term health. Waking up with the sun helps synchronize your circadian rhythm, leading to a cascade of health benefits. Aligning your morning with natural light is one of the simplest yet most powerful strategies to regulate your biology at its core. Early exposure to sunlight activates your circadian rhythm, supporting hormone balance, energy metabolism, cognitive function, and emotional stability. When you align your wake-up time with the natural light of dawn, your body's internal clock becomes more attuned to the natural day-night cycle. This isn't just about getting out of bed; it's about activating your body's internal blueprint for resilience, vitality, and flow. This synchronization can enhance the quality of your sleep, boost your mood, and improve your overall wellbeing. When you rise with the rhythms of nature, you are not just waking up; you are aligning with the systems that keep you well. By tuning in to the sun's schedule, you set the stage for a healthier, more balanced lifestyle. Each sunrise offers a reset and a fresh start filled with possibility, presence, and the power to choose how you show up for your SUPERWELL life.

## MOOD BOOSTER

Basking in natural light can work wonders for your mood. It boosts serotonin levels, like a burst of sunshine for your soul. When you soak up the sun's golden rays, your body releases this feel-good neurotransmitter, lifting your spirits and infusing your day with a radiant sense of wellbeing. This simple yet powerful connection to sunlight acts like nature's own mood enhancer, transforming the everyday into a brighter, more cheerful experience.

## IMPROVED SLEEP

Waking naturally with the rising sun and exposing yourself to morning sunlight within the first 30–60 minutes of being awake helps regulate your circadian rhythm, optimizing both sleep quality and daytime energy. Natural light signals your master clock—called the suprachiasmatic nucleus (SCN)—a small region in the brain that governs your body's internal timing. It cues the body to suppress melatonin and boost cortisol in a balanced way, promoting sustained energy without artificial stimulants. This alignment with light cycles enhances sleep efficiency, cognitive function, and metabolic health, ensuring deeper, more restorative rest at night and a refreshed, energized start to each day.

## HORMONAL BALANCE

Aligning with natural light and dark cycles is essential for hormonal homeostasis, directly influencing key regulators like cortisol, melatonin, and serotonin. Exposure to morning sunlight within the first hour of waking signals the hypothalamus to synchronize the body's circadian rhythm, ensuring a proper cortisol awakening response (CAR)—a crucial factor in energy, metabolism, and stress resilience. This early light exposure also stimulates serotonin production, the precursor to melatonin, supporting mood stability, restful sleep, and optimal endocrine function. By syncing with natural light patterns, the body engages in a biological rhythm that enhances vitality, mental clarity, and long-term metabolic health.

## IMPROVED ENERGY LEVEL

Exposure to natural light in the morning can significantly enhance your alertness and energy levels throughout the day. By starting your day with the invigorating glow of sunlight, you kickstart your body's internal clock, which helps boost your overall wakefulness and vitality. This morning light not only sharpens your focus but also sets a positive tone for the rest of the day, ensuring you stay energized and engaged as you move through your daily activities.

# SUPERWELL TAKEAWAYS

*Natural Awakening & Morning Sunlight:*
*The Foundation of Hormonal Balance*

---

### SUNLIGHT: YOUR DAILY DOSE OF MOOD & METABOLIC MAGIC

- Fifteen minutes of morning sunlight triggers the release of serotonin, the precursor to melatonin, lifting mood and enhancing emotional resilience for the entire day.

- Sunlight exposure reduces the risk of seasonal affective disorder (SAD) by up to 40%, supporting mental clarity and emotional stability.

- Natural light exposure early in the day optimizes dopamine levels, improving motivation, focus, and cognitive performance.

### SUNLIGHT: YOUR BIOLOGICAL POWER SOURCE

- Morning light regulates your circadian rhythm, reinforcing the body's master clock (SCN), which governs everything from metabolism to immune function.

- Early exposure to blue-enriched sunlight suppresses melatonin during the day, ensuring a strong nighttime melatonin pulse for deeper, more restorative sleep.

- Sunlight triggers the release of endorphins, increasing energy, lowering stress hormones, and boosting overall vitality.

## YOUR BODY RUNS ON A CLOCK— STOP BREAKING IT

- Waking up and sleeping at random times disrupts cortisol and melatonin production, leading to chronic fatigue, metabolic dysfunction, and poor sleep quality.
- Circadian rhythm alignment enhances mitochondrial function, optimizing energy production at a cellular level for better endurance and faster recovery.
- Consistent wake-up times strengthen the body's hormonal rhythm, stabilizing insulin sensitivity, reducing inflammation, and promoting longevity.

### SUPERWELL ACTION STEP

Prioritize morning light within 30–60 minutes of waking—unfiltered, outdoors, and without sunglasses to lock in your body's natural rhythm, amplify energy, and lay the foundation for optimal hormonal balance and vitality.

---

## THE SUPERWELL METHOD SHOWS YOU THAT SLOWING DOWN IS *the key to leveling up.*

---

# GROUNDING RITUAL

Sometimes the most powerful wellness tools are the simplest (bonus: *free*) and right beneath your feet. Grounding, or earthing, is the practice of physically connecting your body to the earth's natural surface: barefoot in the grass, standing in sand, or walking on soil. It's more than a calming ritual; it's a biologically restorative act backed by science. The earth carries a subtle negative charge, and when we connect with it directly, we absorb free electrons that reduce inflammation, rebalance stress hormones, and support cellular repair. This isn't just about feeling good in the moment; it's about restoring your internal electrical system to its most natural, healing state. Grounding reminds us that we are nature . . . wired to recharge, reset, and restore. Step outside, plant your feet, and remember that every moment you spend rooted to the earth is an opportunity to come home to yourself—calmer, stronger, and more resilient than before.

## INFLAMMATION REDUCTION

Grounding is like tapping into nature's own healing energy, where the earth's surface gifts you with soothing electrons that tackle inflammation head-on. When you connect barefoot with the ground, these electrons dance into your body, neutralizing pesky free radicals that fuel inflammation. This natural exchange not only calms inflammation but also nurtures your overall health, making grounding a simple yet magical way to boost your wellbeing.

## IMPROVED SLEEP

Regular grounding can significantly enhance both the quality and duration of your sleep. By connecting with the earth's surface, you help stabilize your body's internal rhythms and reduce stress, which can lead to deeper, more restful slumber. This natural practice promotes a more balanced sleep cycle, allowing you to wake up feeling refreshed and revitalized.

## STRESS REDUCTION

Connecting with the earth's energy has a soothing effect on stress levels. When you engage in grounding practices, the natural flow of electrons from the earth helps to calm your nervous system and reduce the impact of stress. This simple yet profound connection with nature promotes a sense of tranquility and balance, helping to alleviate daily tension and foster a more relaxed state of mind.

## ENHANCE IMMUNITY

Grounding supercharges your immune system by harmonizing your body's bioelectrical environment. By connecting with the earth's surface, you invite a stream of balancing electrons that fine-tune your body's electrical rhythms. This natural boost enhances your immune defenses, making grounding a vibrant way to fortify your health and resilience.

## PAIN REDUCTION

Studies reveal that grounding can alleviate chronic pain and enhance overall wellbeing. By connecting with the earth's surface, you tap into its natural energy, which helps ease discomfort and promote a greater sense of health and vitality.

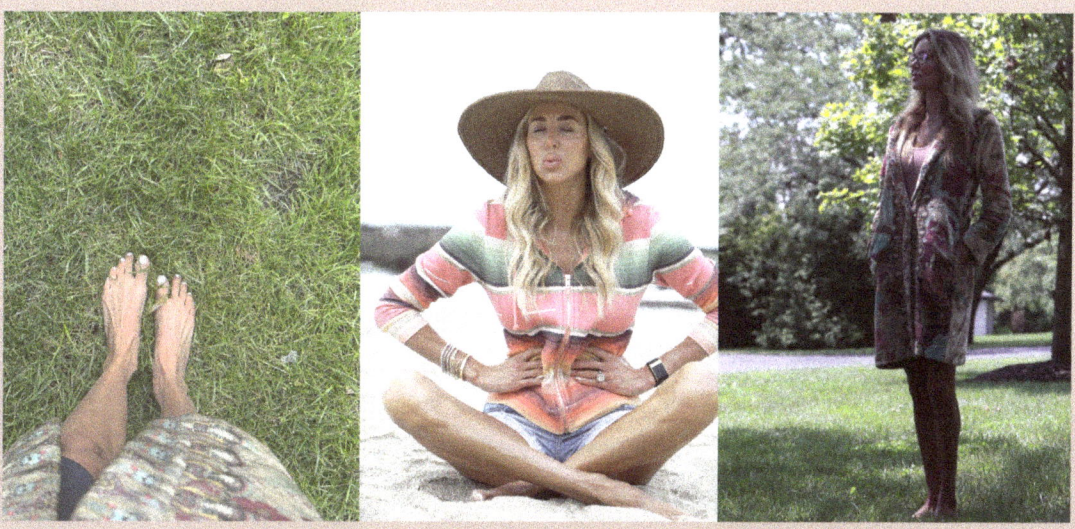

# ACTIVITIES TO CONNECT WITH NATURE

### FOREST BATHING
### *(SHINRIN YOKU)*

- This is a practice of immersing yourself in the atmosphere of the forest by walking slowly, breathing deeply, and engaging your senses.
- Benefit: Relieves stress and improves mental clarity.

### GROUNDING OR EARTHING

- Walk barefoot on grass, sand, or soil.
- Benefit: Reduces inflammation, promotes better sleep, and restores energy balance.

### HIKING & NATURE WALKS

- Explore trails in parks, forests, or nature reserves.
- Benefit: Enhances cardiovascular health, boosts mood, and improves mental focus.

### OUTDOOR YOGA OR MEDITATION

- Practice yoga or meditate in a natural environment to ground yourself and achieve mindfulness.
- Benefit: Promotes mental clarity, reduces stress, and enhances physical flexibility.

### GARDENING OR PLANTING

- Spend time planting, tending to, or simply being around plants.
- Benefit: Reduces anxiety, boosts mood, and improves focus.

## SUPERWELL TAKEAWAYS:

*Grounding Ritual*

---

### GROUNDING = INSTANT ANTI-INFLAMMATORY

- Chronic inflammation is the root of nearly 90% of modern diseases, including heart disease, autoimmune disorders, and neurodegenerative conditions.

- Grounding activates your parasympathetic nervous system, helping to lower inflammation by reducing pro-inflammatory cytokines and oxidative stress.

- Studies show grounding can reduce markers of inflammation in just 30 minutes of direct skin-to-earth contact.

### BETTER SLEEP & NERVOUS SYSTEM REBALANCING

- Sleeping grounded (using a grounding mat or spending time barefoot daily) helps regulate circadian rhythms, leading to deeper, more restorative sleep.

- Grounding has been found to reduce nighttime cortisol spikes by up to 50%, allowing your body to transition more easily into restorative, deep sleep cycles.

- Direct contact with the earth enhances melatonin production, supporting a natural sleep-wake cycle for improved mood, focus, and energy during the day.

## STRESS & ANXIETY REGULATION – YOUR BUILT IN RESET BUTTON

- Grounding lowers stress by stabilizing heart rate variability (HRV), reducing blood pressure, and shifting the body out of fight-or-flight mode.
- Direct contact with the earth has been shown to reduce anxiety and depression symptoms by promoting the release of serotonin and dopamine, nature's built-in mood stabilizers.
- Grounding activates alpha brain waves, the same calming frequency produced during meditation, fostering a state of relaxation and clarity.

## IMMUNE BOOST & PAIN REDUCTION

- Grounding enhances immune function by reducing oxidative stress and regulating inflammatory responses, creating an optimal environment for cellular repair.
- Studies show grounding reduces muscle soreness and speeds up recovery by decreasing white blood cell count and creatine kinase levels, both markers of muscle damage.
- Electrons from the earth neutralize excess positive charges in the body, reducing chronic pain and inflammation without medications or interventions.

## SUPERWELL ACTION STEP

Start your morning grounding ritual by spending 10–15 minutes barefoot outdoors, whether it's on grass, sand, or soil. If getting outside isn't an option, grounding mats and sheets can replicate these benefits indoors.

Your body is designed to sync with the earth's energy, so let it recharge, recalibrate, and bring you back to a state of optimal balance and resilience.

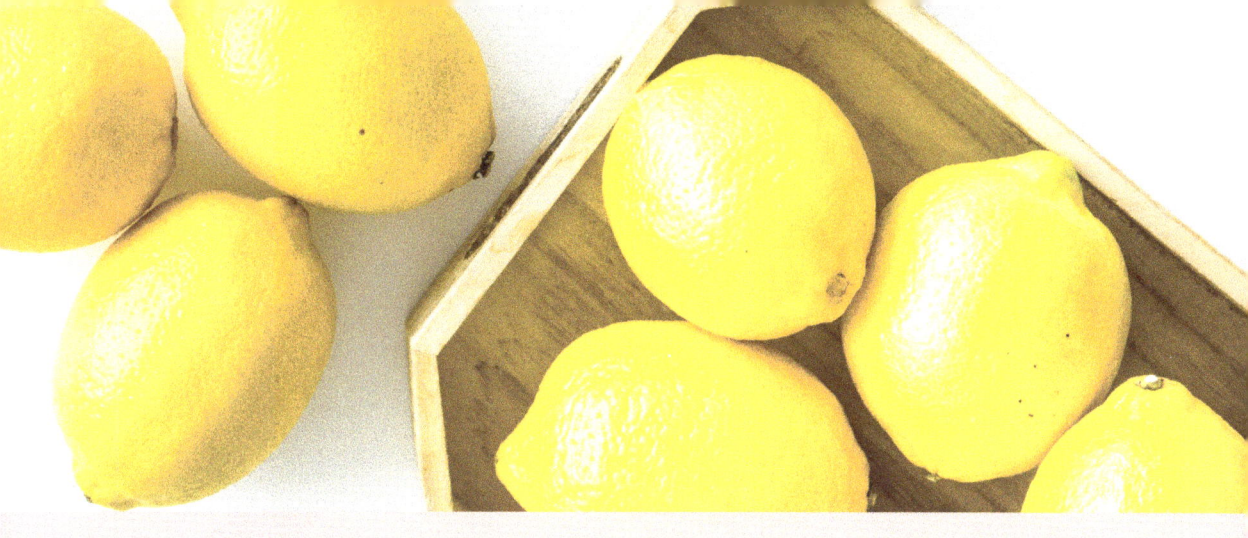

SUPERWELL

# MORNING GUT ELIXIR

### *Your Daily Digestive Reset + Energy Blueprint*

If your gut isn't functioning properly, nothing else in your body can operate at its best. That is why the very first thing I consume each morning is my SUPERWELL Morning Gut Elixir, a foundational part of my daily blueprint for resilience, energy, and digestive wellbeing.

Your gut is more than just a digestive system; it's a command center. It regulates mood, supports brain health, controls inflammation, and houses nearly 70% of your immune system. Even more remarkable is that over 90% of your serotonin—the neurotransmitter that governs happiness and emotional balance—is produced in the gut. So, how you treat your gut sets the tone not just for digestion, but for your mental clarity, energy, and emotional stability.

After 10–12 hours of overnight fasting, your gut lining is especially receptive to nutrients. That is why the *first thing you put in your body matters*. The SUPERWELL Morning Gut Elixir is specifically designed to nourish your gut lining, promote microbiome balance, support liver detox, and fire up your metabolic engine—all before your first bite of food.

## WHY IT WORKS

- **Apple cider vinegar** stimulates stomach acid production, supporting healthy digestion and nutrient absorption while balancing blood sugar to avoid spikes and promoting insulin sensitivity.
- **Lemon juice** floods your body with vitamin C and phytonutrients, supporting collagen production, liver function, and immune defense.
- **L-glutamine** works to repair the gut lining and improve intestinal permeability (goodbye leaky gut).
- **Zen Basil seeds,** rich in prebiotic fiber and omega-3s, gently scrub and soothe the gut, promoting regularity and sweeping out pathogens.
- **Himalayan sea salt** helps replenish trace minerals and balance electrolytes for better hydration.
- **Greens powder** loads your cells with antioxidants, chlorophyll, vitamins, and minerals to kickstart detoxification and energize the body at the cellular level.
- **Filtered water** ensures you are rehydrating your body after sleep while carrying this nutrient-dense blend into every system that needs it.

## THE REAL ENERGY SECRET

This isn't about caffeine crashes or quick fixes: It's about fueling from the inside out. When your gut is nourished and your digestion runs smoothly, your body extracts more energy from the foods you eat, supports mitochondrial function, and reduces inflammatory fatigue. Translation? More energy, fewer cravings, better focus, and a lighter, clearer body and mind.

This one-minute morning ritual is my non-negotiable, and it primes my digestive fire, stabilizes my blood sugar, and keeps my gut-brain axis humming.

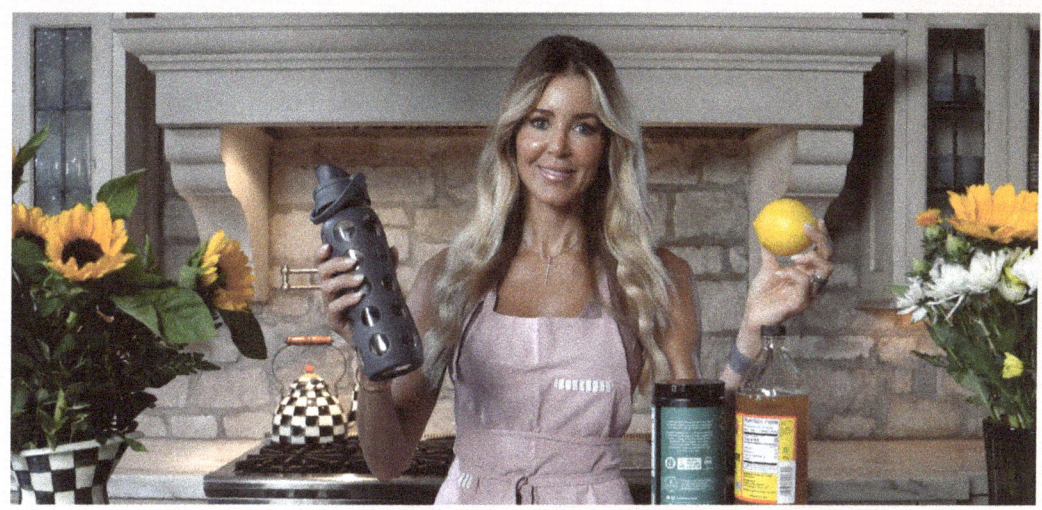

# Morning Gut Elixir

- 1 tablespoon apple cider vinegar (ACV)
- 1 tablespoon Zen Basil seeds, soaked (see note)
- Juice of 1/2 lemon (or pre-made lemon ice cube, see page 41)
- Dash of Himalayan sea salt
- 1 tablespoon greens powder
- 1 teaspoon L-glutamine powder
- 8–12 oz filtered water

1. Combine all ingredients in your favorite glass bottle.
2. Shake vigorously until everything is mixed.

## PRO TIPS

Prep it the night before and leave it on your bathroom sink for an effortless morning routine.

This elixir is your daily reset, setting the tone for a day of SUPERWELL Living. Cheers to vibrant health and a happy gut!

Sip your morning gut elixir with a straw to protect your tooth enamel.

Soaking is key to the success of cooking with Zen Basil seeds and letting them work their wellness magic for the gut. The seeds need to be measured dry and then soaked in water for as little as 10 minutes, or as long as overnight, for them to expand. I recommend keeping a sealed container of fully soaked seeds in your refrigerator; they keep for up to 3–4 days.

SUPERWELL RECIPES

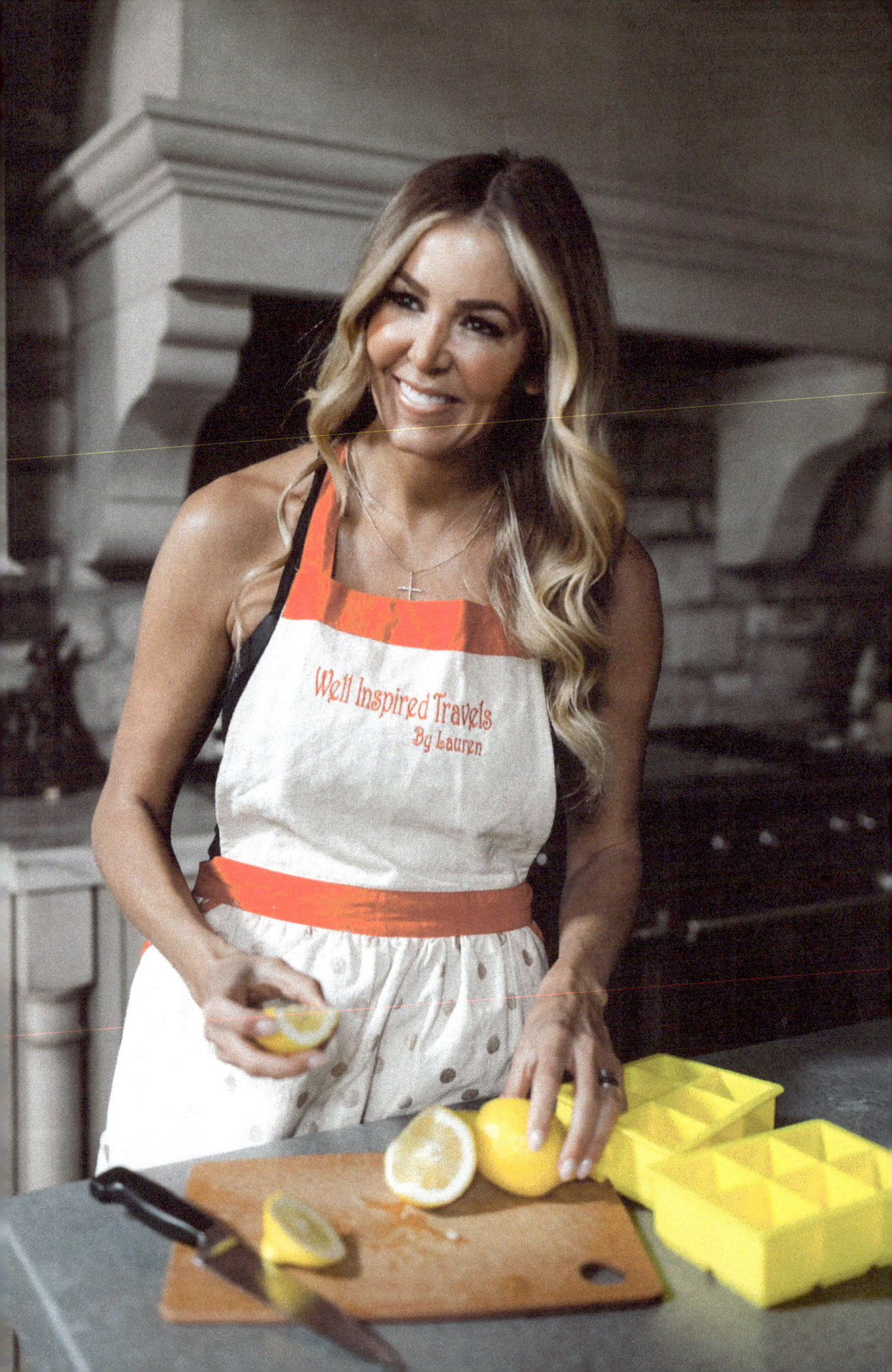

# SUPERWELL WELLNESS ICE CUBES

This is an easy, everyday wellness upgrade. These nutrient-packed frozen cubes support digestion, reduce inflammation, and boost immunity, without any fuss. Just drop one into your morning warm water, bone broth, tea, or gut elixir and sip your way to better energy, skin, and glow. Prep once (my day is Sundays), feel the benefits all week. Keep a variety of these in your freezer and grab based on your body's needs. They are functional, fast, and packed with flavor—your morning just got a SUPERWELL upgrade!

## BASIC LEMON BOOST CUBES

1/2 cup fresh-squeezed lemon juice

1/2 cup filtered water

1. Whisk lemon juice and water together. Pour into silicone ice cube trays and freeze. Once solid, store in a sealed container or freezer bag.

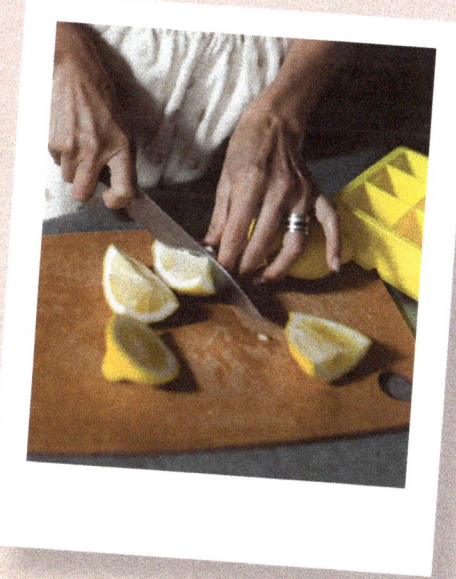

### WHY IT'S SUPERWELL APPROVED

✔ Alkalizing and rich in vitamin C, lemon boosts digestion, supports liver detox, and hydrates at a cellular level, making it the ideal foundation for your morning ritual.

## GINGER-TURMERIC-LEMON CUBES WITH BLACK PEPPER

2 tablespoons freshly grated ginger

2 tablespoons freshly grated turmeric

1/2 cup fresh-squeezed lemon juice

1/8 teaspoon black pepper
   (to enhance curcumin absorption)

1/2 cup filtered water

1. Blend all ingredients until smooth. Pour into silicone ice cube trays and freeze. Once solid, store in a sealed container or freezer bag.

### WHY IT'S SUPERWELL APPROVED

✔ Anti-inflammatory and immune-boosting, these golden cubes help regulate blood sugar, calm inflammation, and jumpstart digestion. Black pepper is key for curcumin bioavailability. Without it, turmeric isn't fully absorbed.

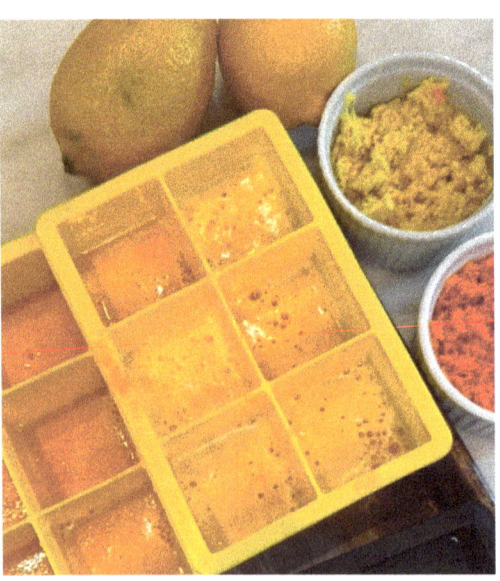
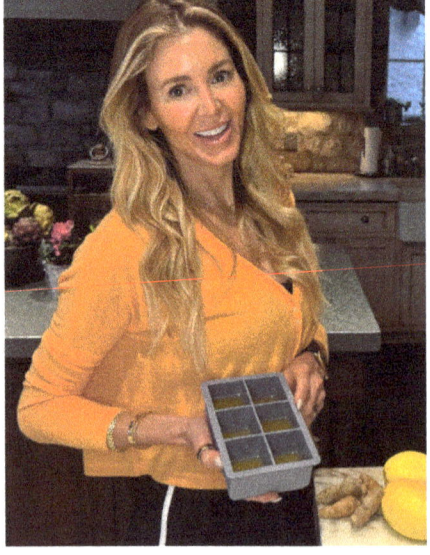

## LEMON-GINGER CUBES

2 tablespoons freshly grated ginger

1/2 cup fresh-squeezed lemon juice

1/2 cup filtered water

1. Blend ingredients until well combined. Pour into silicone ice cube trays and freeze. Once solid, store in a sealed container or freezer bag.

### WHY IT'S SUPERWELL APPROVED

✔ This classic combo soothes the stomach, reduces bloating, and revs up digestion while supporting immune resilience. It's a warm tonic go-to.

## STRAIGHT GINGER CUBES

1/4 cup freshly grated or blended ginger

3/4 cup filtered water

1. Blend until smooth. Pour into silicone ice cube trays and freeze. Once solid, store in a sealed container or freezer bag.

### WHY IT'S SUPERWELL APPROVED

✔ These have pure ginger power—excellent for nausea, inflammation, and immune defense. Add to warm water, bone broth, tea, or soup for an instant gut-loving boost.

## SUPERWELL SIGNATURE
# Bone Broth

A mineral-rich, collagen-packed, deeply nourishing broth infused with functional herbs and veggies to support your glow, gut, and grounding.

**YIELD: ABOUT 10 CUPS**

- 2–3 pounds grass-fed beef bones (with marrow and knuckles) or organic pasture-raised chicken bones (backs, necks, wings, or feet)
- 1 chicken foot or 1 small beef tendon (optional, for extra gelatin!)
- 2 carrots, chopped
- 2 celery stalks, chopped
- 1 onion, quartered (skin on for color and minerals)
- 1 bulb garlic, halved crosswise
- 1-inch fresh ginger root, sliced
- 1-inch fresh turmeric root, sliced
- 1 bay leaf
- 1 teaspoon black peppercorns
- 1 strip kombu seaweed (optional, adds trace minerals and umami)

### Optional Herbal Glow Twist:

- A few sprigs of favorite herbs, like fresh thyme and rosemary
- 1 tablespoon dried nettle or dandelion root (supports liver and skin)
- 1 star anise or cinnamon stick (optional, adds subtle warmth and depth)
- 12 cups filtered water (or enough to cover)
- 2 tablespoons apple cider vinegar (helps pull minerals from bones)

1. Prep the bones (optional but recommended). Roast bones in the oven at 400°F for 20–25 minutes until golden. This deepens the flavor and gives a richer color.

2. Add all ingredients to a large stockpot or slow cooker. Pour in filtered water to cover (about 12 cups). Let sit for 30 minutes before heating. This gives the vinegar time to help extract minerals from the bones.

3. Bring to a simmer, then reduce to low and cook. If cooking on a stovetop, simmer gently for 12–24 hours. Add more water as needed to keep the pot from drying out. If using a slow cooker, set on low for 24 hours. Skim foam if needed in the first hour.

4. Strain the broth through a fine mesh strainer. Discard solids. Let cool, then store in glass jars or ice cube trays. Refrigerate for up to 5 days or freeze for up to 3 months.

5. Reheat gently and enjoy solo, or use it as a base for soups, risottos, or grain cooking water.

## SUPERWELL APPROVED

✔ Collagen and gelatin support skin elasticity, gut lining, and joint health.

✔ Turmeric, ginger, and garlic calm inflammation and boost immunity.

✔ Seaweed and herbs add trace minerals and liver support.

✔ Nettle and dandelion root enhance detox and radiance from within.

# SUPERWELL SERVING SUGGESTIONS

**Sip warm in the morning with a pinch of sea salt and a squeeze of lemon.**

**Blend with 1 teaspoon of coconut oil + a dash of cayenne for a spicy morning jumpstart.**

**Stir in collagen peptides for an extra protein punch.**

**Add a spoonful of miso once warmed (never boil miso) for probiotic benefits.**

# 5 SUPERWELL GUT HEALTH FACTS

## 1. YOUR GUT IS YOUR IMMUNE SYSTEM'S HQ

- 70% of your immune system resides in your gut, acting as the first line of defense against harmful invaders.
- A strong gut barrier prevents toxins, pathogens, and undigested food particles from entering your bloodstream, reducing chronic inflammation.
- A compromised gut can trigger autoimmune conditions, allergies, and systemic inflammation.

## 2. YOUR GUT INFLUENCES YOUR MOOD

- 90% of serotonin, the "feel-good" neurotransmitter, is produced in your gut, directly impacting mood, stress response, and mental clarity.
- A disrupted gut microbiome is linked to anxiety, depression, and brain fog, emphasizing the gut-brain connection.
- Supporting gut health through fiber, probiotics, and stress reduction can enhance emotional resilience and mental wellbeing.

## 3. DIVERSE GUT BACTERIA = THRIVING HEALTH

- Your gut is home to trillions of microbes, and a diverse microbiome is essential for digestion, immunity, and even metabolic function.
- A high-fiber diet with fermented foods (like sauerkraut, kefir, and kimchi) supports microbial diversity and gut balance.
- Poor gut health has been linked to metabolic disorders, obesity, and neurodegenerative diseases.

## 4. LEAKY GUT = SILENT INFLAMMATION & SYSTEMIC ISSUES

- Leaky gut (i.e., intestinal permeability) occurs when the gut lining is damaged, allowing toxins and undigested food particles to leak into the bloodstream.
- This triggers widespread inflammation, leading to symptoms like bloating, fatigue, joint pain, food sensitivities, and skin issues.
- Healing the gut with collagen, glutamine, prebiotics, and an anti-inflammatory diet can restore the integrity of the gut lining.

## 5. GUT HEALTH = METABOLIC & HORMONAL BALANCE

- Your gut microbiome plays a key role in regulating metabolism, blood sugar, and insulin sensitivity.
- An unhealthy gut is linked to hormonal imbalances, increased cortisol, and difficulty maintaining a healthy weight.
- Prioritizing gut health supports efficient digestion, energy production, and balanced hormone levels.

### SUPERWELL ACTION STEP

Nurture your gut daily with whole foods, hydration, stress management, and microbiome-friendly nutrients to support longevity, energy, and total-body wellness.

# SUPPLEMENT STACK

As you savor your SUPERWELL Morning Gut Elixir, consider completing your ritual with a few key supplements—if they align with your individual needs. Personally, I'm not a huge fan of loading up on endless pills and powders. I believe in getting the majority of my vitamins and minerals from real, whole, nutrient-dense foods. That said, there are a few well-chosen supplements I value for targeted support.

Probiotics help maintain a balanced gut microbiome, high-quality fish oil delivers essential omega-3s for brain and heart health, and other supplements can enhance cellular resilience and recovery. Always consult with your doctor or medical provider before beginning any new supplement regimen. When used intentionally, these tools can help reinforce your wellness blueprint and set a strong foundation for the day ahead.

## GUT HEALTH

Probiotics are key to maintaining a healthy gut microbiome, which is essential for effective digestion and strong immunity. By fostering beneficial bacteria and keeping harmful microbes at bay, probiotics support nutrient absorption and enhance immune function, contributing to overall wellbeing.

## CELLULAR HEALTH

Certain supplements are specifically designed to enhance cellular health and promote longevity. By providing essential nutrients and antioxidants, these supplements help protect cells from oxidative stress and support their vital functions. This can lead to improved cellular repair, reduced inflammation, and overall better health. Incorporating such supplements into your routine can contribute to longer-lasting vitality and a greater sense of wellbeing.

## BRAIN FUNCTION

Omega-3s are essential for boosting cognitive function and reducing brain fog. These fatty acids improve brain health by enhancing communication between neurons and reducing inflammation, leading to better mental clarity and sharper focus.

## HEART HEALTH

Omega-3s are crucial for cardiovascular health, as they reduce inflammation, lower triglycerides, and support healthy blood pressure. These fatty acids help maintain a well-functioning heart and reduce the risk of heart disease.

## ANTI-INFLAMMATORY

These supplements collectively work to reduce inflammation, thereby promoting overall wellness. By targeting various inflammatory pathways and supporting the body's natural anti-inflammatory responses, they help alleviate discomfort and support better health. This comprehensive approach contributes to improved vitality, enhances recovery, and supports overall wellbeing.

## GENERAL WELLNESS & ANTI-INFLAMMATORY

- Multivitamin – Ensures a broad spectrum of essential nutrients to fill any gaps in the diet
- Turmeric/Curcumin – Provides anti-inflammatory and antioxidant support
- Omega-3 Fatty Acids (Fish Oil) – Provides essential omega-3 fatty acids for heart health and inflammation reduction
- Collagen Peptides – Promotes skin elasticity, joint health, and hair and nail strength
- Ashwagandha – Adaptogen provides stress relief and hormone balance
- Magnesium (Glycinate or Citrate) – Supports relaxation, muscle function, and sleep

## GUT HEALTH

- Probiotic – Supports a balanced gut microbiome, crucial for optimal digestion and immunity
- L-Glutamine – Aids gut lining repair and supports intestinal health
- Digestive Enzymes – Helps break down food and improve nutrient absorption

## ENERGY & FOCUS

- B Complex Vitamins – Supports energy levels and cognitive function
- Vitamin B12 – Vital for energy production and nerve function
- Lion's Mane Mushroom – Enhances cognitive function and nerve health
- Rhodiola Rosea – Boosts energy, endurance, and mental clarity

## SLEEP & RECOVERY

- Melatonin – Supports sleep cycles and circadian rhythm
- L-Theanine – Promotes relaxation and stress reduction without drowsiness
- Valerian Root – Aids natural sleep and relaxes muscles

## IMMUNE SUPPORT

- Vitamin C – Boosts the immune system and promotes healthy skin
- Vitamin D3 + K2 – Supports bone health, immune function, and mood
- Zinc – Essential for immune support and cellular function
- Elderberry – Known for antiviral and immune-boosting properties

## HORMONAL BALANCE

- Maca Root – Supports hormone regulation and energy
- Chaste Tree (Vitex) – Helps balance hormones and menstrual cycles
- Evening Primrose Oil – Supports skin health and hormonal balance

## PHYSICAL PERFORMANCE & MUSCLE HEALTH

- Creatine – Enhances physical performance and supports muscle health, even for women

Incorporating these supplements helps maintain balance, support the body's needs, and keep you feeling your best every day.

*Always consult your doctor before starting any new vitamins or supplements.

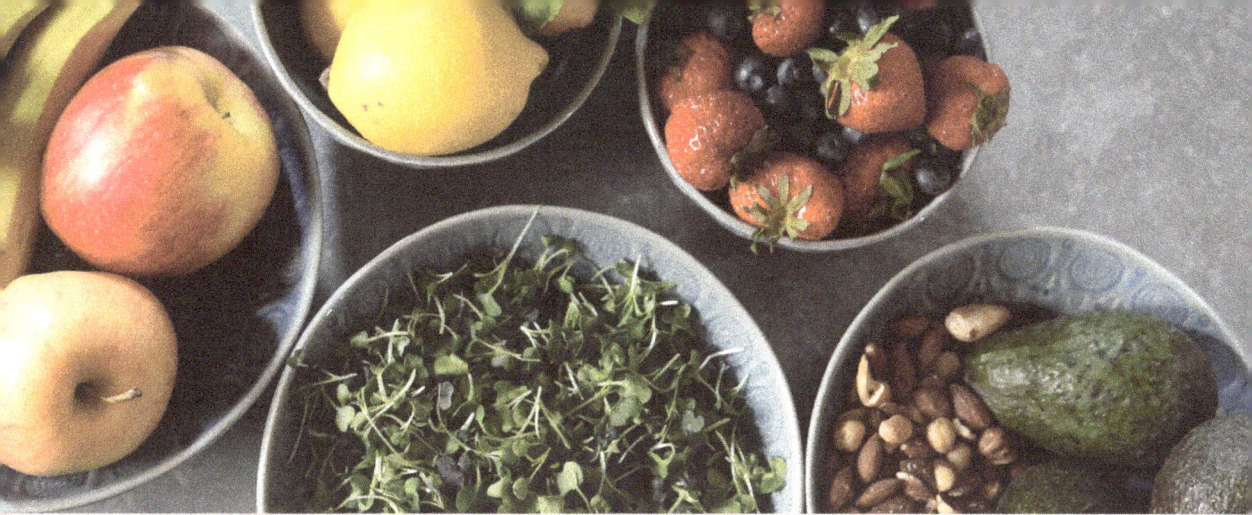

## START STRONG:
# WHY A SAVORY BREAKFAST IS A SUPERWELL NON-NEGOTIABLE

One of the most impactful ways to set the tone for a SUPERWELL day begins with what is on your plate—specifically, your first meal of the morning. "Nourishing Nutrition" is a core pillar of the SUPERWELL Living Method, and you will see its importance woven throughout this book. That's because what you choose to eat (and when and how you eat it) influences everything from your blood sugar and energy levels to your mood, mental clarity, metabolism, and hormone regulation.

Starting your day with a savory, protein-forward breakfast rather than one filled with sugar or refined carbs is one of the most strategic shifts you can make for your health. Why? A savory meal stabilizes blood glucose, reduces the risk of mid-morning crashes, and supports optimal metabolic function. Unlike sugary cereals, juices, pastries, or even sweetened smoothies that can spike insulin and send you into a rollercoaster of cravings and fatigue, a balanced savory breakfast helps regulate your hunger hormones (like ghrelin and leptin) and keeps your energy consistent throughout the day.

To maximize blood sugar balance and satiety, it's also important to *eat in the right order*:

1. Start with fiber-rich greens or vegetables.
2. Follow with quality protein.
3. Then, include healthy fats.
4. Add a clean, complex carbohydrate if desired, especially if you are preparing for a physically demanding day or heading into an intense workout. These healthy carbs (like sweet potatoes, quinoa, sourdough bread, or root vegetables) provide sustainable fuel without the crash, supporting glycogen replenishment and endurance.

This order of operations supports digestive efficiency, slows the glucose response, and minimizes post-meal inflammation or crashes. You will see throughout the SUPERWELL blueprint that small, strategic shifts like these are what create sustainable transformation.

A savory, nutrient-dense breakfast isn't just a meal—it's your morning fuel, your metabolic ignition switch, and your first step toward living SUPERWELL. Let's get into the *how*.

---

THE BEAUTY OF THE SUPERWELL
METHOD IS IN ITS SIMPLICITY —
*small shifts, big impact.*

---

### HOW TO BUILD
# THE ULTIMATE SAVORY BREAKFAST PLATE

A savory, blood sugar–balanced breakfast isn't just about what's on your plate; it's about *how* you eat it and why. By focusing on nutrient synergy and proper food sequencing, you can support your metabolism, hormonal health, energy regulation, and digestive ease, all before 9 A.M.

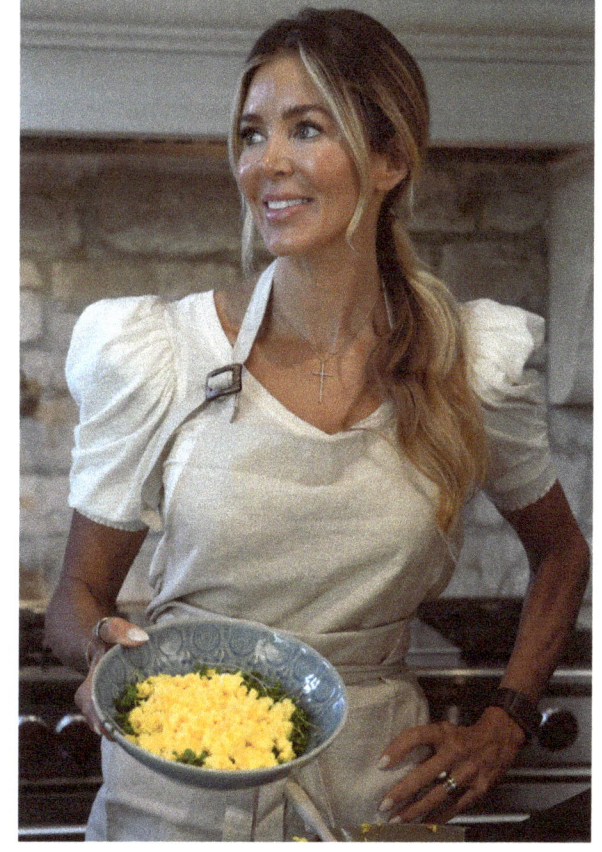

Here's how to structure your SUPERWELL breakfast plate for optimal nourishment and performance:

## 1. START WITH FIBER-RICH VEGGIES

Begin your meal with non-starchy vegetables like leafy greens (spinach, arugula), microgreens, zucchini, mushrooms, tomatoes, or sautéed broccoli. These provide prebiotic fiber to feed your gut microbiome and act as a glucose "shield," slowing the absorption of sugars and starches that follow. Starting with fiber helps blunt post-meal blood sugar spikes and supports digestion.

## 2. FOLLOW WITH HIGH-QUALITY PROTEIN

Next, add a protein anchor to your plate. Think pasture-raised eggs, wild-caught salmon, organic turkey sausage, or a clean protein shake (ideally 20–30 g per meal). Protein is the most satiating macronutrient; it balances blood sugar, curbs cravings, supports lean muscle maintenance, and provides critical amino acids for mood, repair, and energy production.

## 3. LAYER IN HEALTHY FATS

Fats provide satiety, support hormone production, and enhance nutrient absorption (especially fat-soluble vitamins A, D, E, and K). Add half an avocado, drizzle with extra virgin olive oil, or sprinkle in raw seeds like pumpkin or hemp. You can also cook with grass-fed ghee or avocado oil for heat-stable options.

## 4. OPTIONAL: END WITH A CLEAN CARB (IF NEEDED)

If your morning includes a workout, long walk, or you are heading into a physically or cognitively demanding day, consider a small portion of complex carbohydrates at the *end* of your meal. Options include roasted sweet potatoes, sourdough bread, root vegetables, quinoa, black beans, or steel-cut oats. This sequencing helps control the glycemic impact and gives you lasting energy without the crash.

## 5. AVOID SUGAR-LOADED PITFALLS

Skip refined grains, pastries, juices, dried fruits, and sweetened yogurts or granolas. These spike insulin, crash your energy mid-morning, and dysregulate hunger hormones. Whole fruit is optional, but if included, treat it as your carb and eat it last, after protein and fiber.

## SUPERWELL Pro Tips

✔ **Batch Prep:** Roast a tray of vegetables and protein at dinner to repurpose into a warm, savory breakfast the next morning. Add greens and an egg, and you are done. Leftovers for the SUPERWELL win!

✔ **Keep It Simple:** A few quality ingredients are more powerful than an overcomplicated meal. Think: arugula + eggs + olive oil + leftover roasted sweet potatoes = balanced brilliance.

✔ **Make It Yours:** Your savory plate is one of your most powerful tools in your wellness blueprint. Adjust it to your goals, your day, and your body's cues.

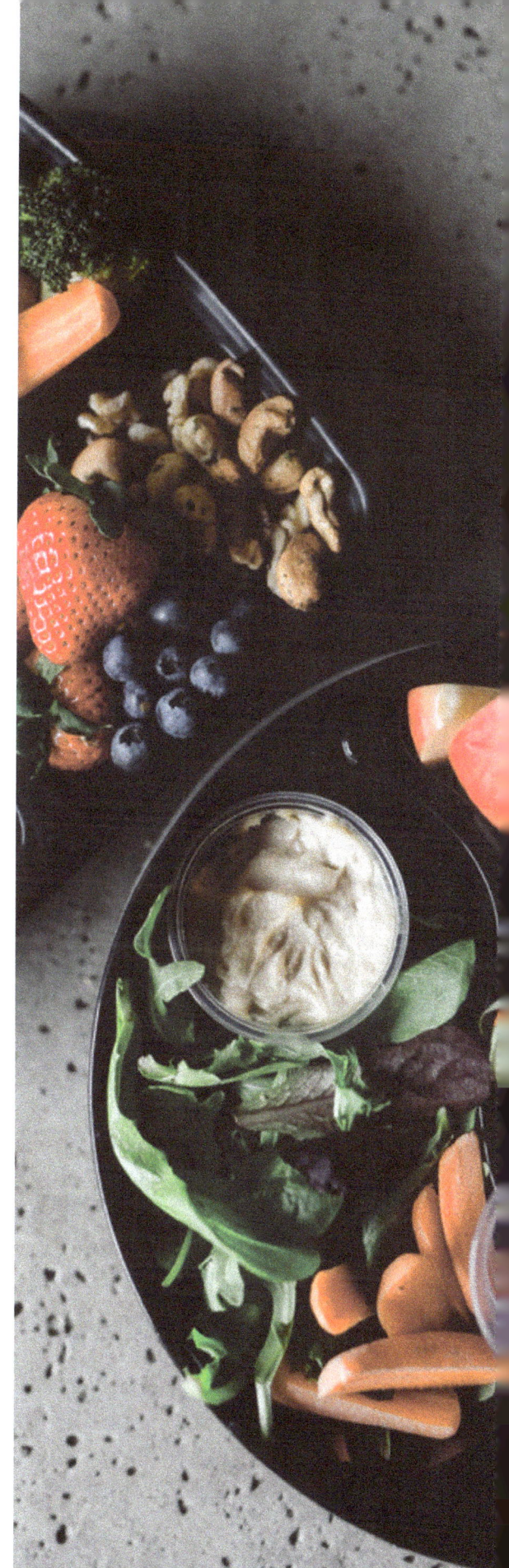

## SUPERWELL
# BREAKFAST FAVORITES

### MAGIC MATCHA ZEN BASIL SEED PUDDING

This recipe is a calm energy reset you can prep ahead for mornings, mid-day slumps, or mindful moments of self-care. This pudding is packed with adaptogens, healthy fats, antioxidants, and natural fiber to support digestion, glowing skin, blood sugar balance, and long-lasting energy. Think of it as a glow-up meets brain boost in one delicious spoonful.

**YIELD: 2 SERVINGS**

- 1/4 cup Zen Basil seeds
- 1/3 cup filtered water
- 1 cup unsweetened almond milk or coconut milk or milk of choice
- 1-1/2 tablespoons full-fat coconut cream
- 1 teaspoon ceremonial grade matcha powder
- 1 tablespoon manuka honey (or sub with maple syrup for vegan version)
- 1/4 teaspoon pure vanilla extract
- Pinch of sea salt (brings all flavors forward)

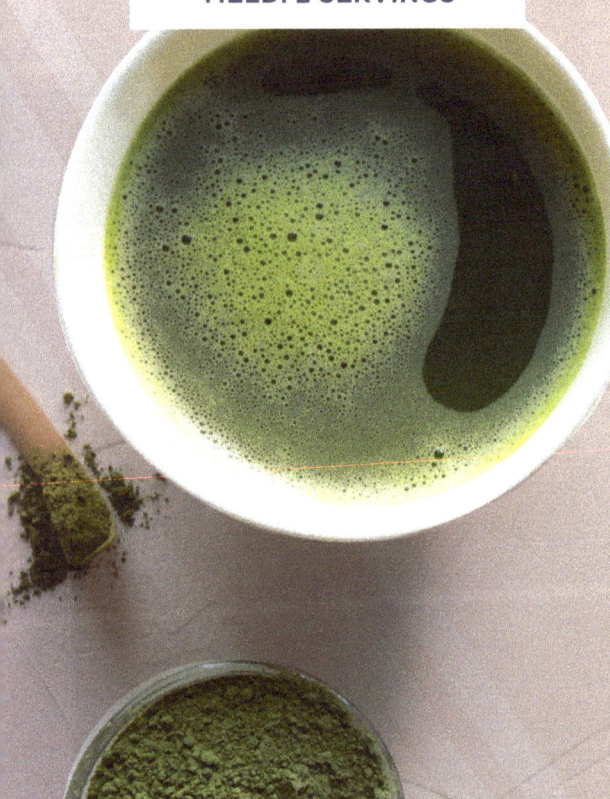

## Breakfast Favorites | 57

### *Optional Super Boosts*

1/2 teaspoon maca powder
(adaptogen, hormone support)

1/4 teaspoon Ceylon cinnamon
(blood sugar balance)

1 tablespoon (1 scoop) collagen powder or plant-based vanilla protein
(for satiety + skin)

### *Toppings* (optional but encouraged)

Fresh sliced strawberries or kiwi
(for vitamin C + color)

Toasted coconut flakes

Raw pistachios or chopped walnuts

Drizzle of extra manuka honey or coconut yogurt

Sprinkle sesame or hemp seeds for texture and omega-3s

---

1. Soak the basil seeds in the filtered water for at least 20 minutes, or overnight in the fridge for best texture. They'll form a gel-like consistency.
2. In a mixing bowl or blender, whisk together the milk, coconut cream, matcha powder, honey, vanilla, salt, and any optional add-ins until smooth and fully combined. A frother or small whisk works great to blend the matcha.
3. Stir the soaked basil seeds into the mixture until evenly distributed.
4. Pour into jars or an airtight container and refrigerate for at least 2–3 hours or overnight until thickened.
5. Layer with toppings of choice and enjoy chilled. Perfect as a morning ritual, on-the-go snack, or healthy dessert.

---

### WHY IT'S SUPERWELL APPROVED

✔ Zen Basil seeds = fiber, prebiotics, and hydration for gut and skin

✔ Matcha + manuka honey = calm energy, antimicrobial and antioxidant power

✔ Coconut cream = satisfying healthy fats to keep you full and your hormones happy

✔ Optional collagen or protein = strength and glow support in one

## SUPERWELL RECIPES

# SUPERWELL-INSPIRED GREATEST Granola

This crunchy, nourishing classic reimagined for balance, glow, and blood sugar support. This isn't your average granola; it's a nutrient-dense, fiber-rich, blood sugar–conscious powerhouse crafted to keep you energized, satisfied, and supported throughout the day. Every ingredient is intentionally chosen to align with the SUPERWELL philosophy: pairing healthy fats, clean protein, complex carbs, and anti-inflammatory superfoods in one crave-worthy blend.

I have perfected this recipe in our home as a pantry staple, whether it's layered into a yogurt bowl, added to smoothie bowls, or enjoyed by the handful with a matcha latte in hand. It's the kind of granola that leaves you full, not foggy.

This is fuel for your nervous system, skin, and soul; a crunchy reminder that every bite is a chance to nourish and elevate.

- 4 cups gluten-free rolled oats (32-ounce bag)
- 1 cup unsalted crushed pecans
- 1 cup unsalted slivered almonds
- 1/2 cup raw cashews, roughly chopped (creamy texture and mineral-rich)
- 1/2 cup raw sunflower seeds
- 1/4 cup mixed Zen Basil seeds, chia seeds, and ground flaxseeds (optional, for omega-3s and gut-friendly fiber)
- 1 tablespoon ground cinnamon (blood sugar balance and warm flavor)
- 1 teaspoon sea salt
- 1/2 cup melted coconut oil (healthy fat for satiety and skin glow)
- 1/2 cup pure maple syrup (natural sweetener with trace minerals)
- 2 teaspoons vanilla extract

## Optional Post-Bake Add-Ins

- Unsweetened coconut flakes
- Dark chocolate chips
- Dried cherries, goji berries, or mulberries
- Crushed freeze-dried strawberries or raspberries
- A swirl of almond or peanut butter for clusters

1. Preheat oven to 350°F. Place parchment paper on a baking sheet.

2. In a large mixing bowl, toss together the oats, pecans, almonds, cashews, sunflower seeds, optional Zen Basil seed blend, cinnamon, and salt.

3. In a separate bowl, whisk together the melted coconut oil, maple syrup, and vanilla extract. Pour over the dry ingredients and stir until evenly coated.

4. Spread the mixture evenly on the parchment-lined baking sheet. Bake at 350°F for 20 minutes. Remove from the oven and stir well.

5. Let the granola cool completely, about 20–30 minutes. This is when it crisps and forms beautiful clusters. Once cool, break the granola into your preferred texture.

6. Stir in your desired post-bake add-ins. Store in an airtight container for up to 2 weeks or longer if refrigerated.

## WHY IT'S SUPERWELL APPROVED

✔ Balanced macronutrients for blood sugar stability and satiety

✔ Cashews + nuts provide magnesium and healthy fats for stress resilience

✔ Coconut oil + cinnamon support hormone balance and digestion

✔ Customizable to align with your nutritional needs and cravings

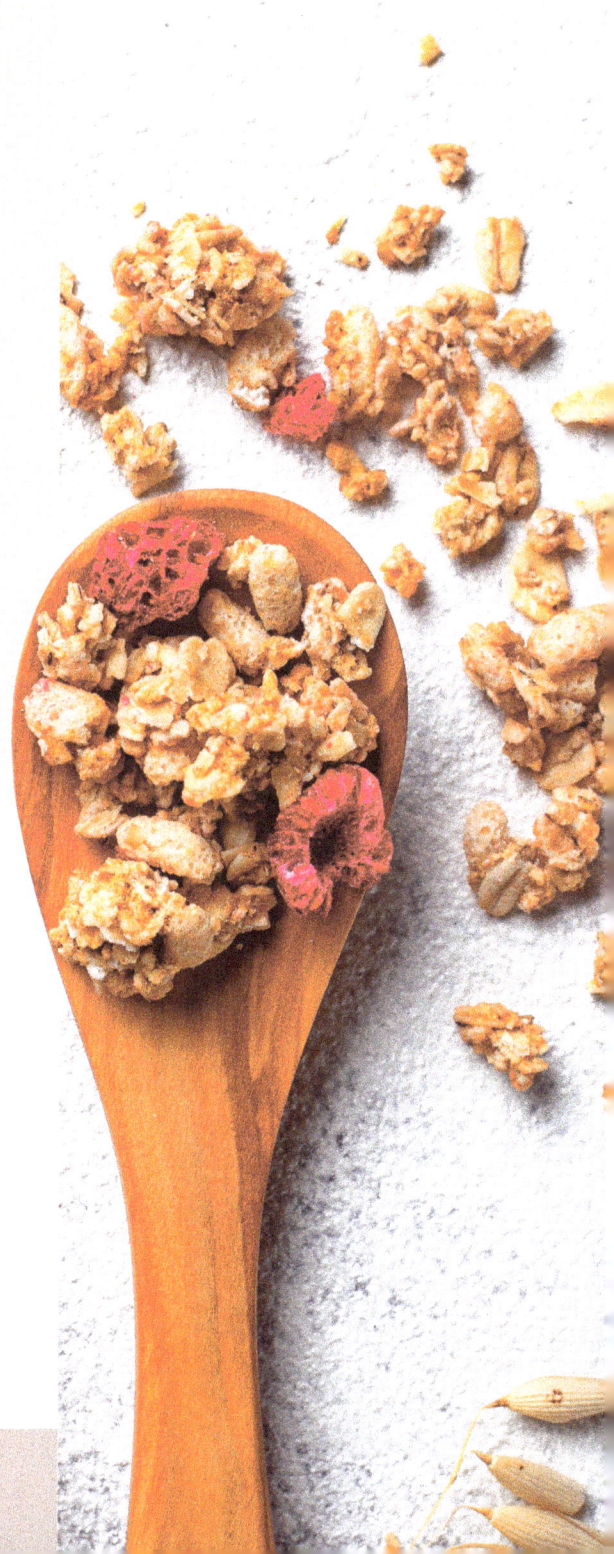

# SUPERWELL
# Egg White Bites

## THE CORE RECIPE + CUSTOM VARIATIONS

*Your High-Protein, Blood Sugar-Friendly Power Bites*

These protein-packed egg white bites are a staple in the SUPERWELL kitchen, quick to prep, easy to store, and ideal for stabilizing blood sugar and fueling your morning with clean, anti-inflammatory energy. Each bite delivers a balance of high-quality protein, healthy fats, and micronutrient-rich vegetables, supporting metabolic health, hormone balance, and satiety without spiking glucose.

Perfect as a grab-and-go breakfast, a post-workout snack, or even a savory mid-afternoon pick-me-up, this recipe is highly customizable so you never get bored. Make a batch on Sunday, and you are set for the week with a SUPERWELL habit that takes the guesswork out of your morning routine.

**YIELD: 12 BITES**

- 1 tablespoon olive or avocado oil
- 1 bunch asparagus, sliced
- 1/2 cup mushrooms, sliced
- 1/2 teaspoon sea salt
- 1 carton (16 ounces) egg whites
- 1 cup full-fat Greek yogurt (adds protein and creaminess)
- 1 cup grated Gruyère or cheese of choice (optional, for richness and flavor)

*Optional Add-Ins:*

- Cracked black pepper
- Everything but bagel spice
- Pinch of garlic powder
- Fresh herbs, like dill or chives, minced

1. Preheat oven to 375°F. Line a 12-cup muffin tin with parchment liners or silicone baking cups.

2. Heat olive oil in a skillet over medium heat. Sauté asparagus and mushrooms with salt for 5–7 minutes until fork-tender. Let cool slightly.

3. In a large bowl, whisk together egg whites, Greek yogurt, and shredded cheese until well combined. Stir in any desired optional add-ins.

4. Fill each muffin cup about three-quarters full with the egg mixture. Spoon the veggie mixture evenly into each cup.

5. Bake for 15–18 minutes, or until the center is set and edges are lightly golden.

6. Let cool for 5 minutes before removing from tin. Store in an airtight container in the fridge for up to 5 days. Reheat in the microwave for 30–45 seconds.

## WHY IT'S SUPERWELL APPROVED

✔ High in protein for satiety, muscle recovery, and hormone support

✔ Blood sugar friendly with no refined carbs or added sugars

✔ Customizable to fit your cravings, goals, or fridge contents

✔ Meal-prep friendly to streamline your mornings

## SUPERWELL VARIATIONS:
*Switch It Up Weekly*

### Mediterranean Glow Bites
Replace Gruyère with feta or goat cheese.

Add cherry tomatoes, kalamata olives, spinach, and a dash of oregano.

### Southwest Savory Bites
Use pepper jack or cheddar.

Add diced bell peppers, red onion, black beans, and cumin or chili powder.

Top with a spoonful of salsa before serving.

### Anti-Inflammatory Power Bites
Use turmeric and curry powder.

Add broccoli, zucchini, and cauliflower rice.

Replace cheese with nutritional yeast for a dairy-free option.

### Green Goddess Detox Bites
Use mozzarella, or skip cheese for a lighter bite.

Add kale, spinach, chopped green onion, and fresh dill or parsley.

Top with a drizzle of pesto when serving.

### Hearty Protein Boost Bites
Add chopped turkey sausage, rotisserie chicken, or smoked salmon.

Include sautéed onions, sweet potato hash, or leeks.

Mix in fresh thyme or rosemary for added flavor.

## PRO TIPS

Use a silicone muffin pan for easy cleanup and perfect release.

Batch-prep different versions in one pan by dividing fillings into sections.

Serve with a side of SUPERWELL Morning Gut Elixir or a savory breakfast salad for a complete, energizing meal.

## SUPERWELL BERRY PROTEIN
# Oat Cup

This creamy layered cup is part breakfast, part antioxidant-powered beauty ritual. With fiber-rich berries, omega-3–loaded basil seeds, and clean protein, it's a delicious way to support glowing skin, balanced blood sugar, and a nourished start to your day. This is the kind of breakfast (or snack!) that keeps you full, energized, and glowing from the inside out.

**YIELD: 1 SERVING**

- 1 tablespoon Zen Basil seeds
- 1/4 cup filtered water
- 1/2 cup instant oats
- 3 large organic strawberries, mashed
- 1/4 cup organic raspberries, mashed
- 2 tablespoons unsweetened coconut yogurt or Greek-style plant-based yogurt
- 2 tablespoons unsweetened vanilla almond milk or milk of choice (add more for blending and desired consistency)
- Dash of vanilla extract
- Salt, to taste
- Stevia or monk fruit, to taste
- 1/2 cup (about 1 scoop) favorite berry protein powder (optional but recommended)

### For the Layers:

- 1/4 cup mashed strawberries and raspberries
- 2 tablespoons melted dark chocolate chips (80%+ cacao)
- 1/2 teaspoon coconut oil

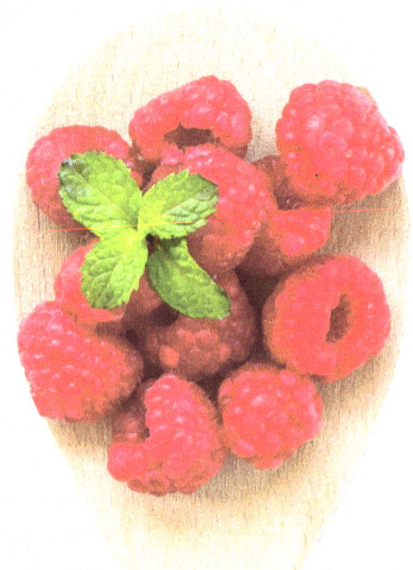

1. Soak the Zen Basil seeds in water for at least 15 minutes.

2. In a blender, combine oats, mashed berries, yogurt, milk, vanilla, salt, sweetener, Zen Basil seeds, and protein powder (if using).

3. Blend until smooth and creamy. Adjust sweetness if needed.

4. In a serving glass or jar, layer the extra mashed strawberries and raspberries at the bottom.

5. Pour the creamy oat mixture on top.

6. Mix together the melted dark chocolate and coconut oil. Drizzle mixture over the top.

7. Let set in the fridge to allow the chocolate to harden and flavors to meld.

## WHY IT'S SUPERWELL APPROVED

✔ Zen Basil seeds are hydration heroes, rich in omega-3s and gut-friendly fiber.

✔ Berries fight inflammation and support glowing skin with vitamin C and polyphenols.

✔ VEGA protein supports muscle repair and hormone health.

✔ Dark chocolate = antioxidants + indulgence, the 80/20 way.

## SUPERWELL STRONG AVOCADO TOAST

This isn't your basic avocado toast—it's fortified with protein, fiber, and healthy fats to keep you strong, sharp, and energized. Ideal for muscle recovery, brain health, and all-day glow, this powerhouse combo is your secret weapon for busy mornings.

**YIELD: 1 SERVING**

- 2 whole organic eggs (optional)
- 2 slices of sourdough bread (or sprouted grain)
- Avocado oil or ghee
- 1/2 ripe avocado, mashed
- 2 tablespoons low-fat Good Culture organic cottage cheese
- Handful of microgreens (like broccoli, arugula, or radish)

### *Optional Toppings*

- Drizzle chili oil
- Manuka honey
- Sprinkle red pepper flakes for kick

1. In a shallow bowl, whisk both eggs until fully combined.
2. Dip each slice of bread into the egg mixture, coating both sides.
3. Heat a skillet over medium heat and lightly grease with avocado oil or ghee.
4. Cook the soaked bread for 2–3 minutes per side, until golden and slightly crispy.
5. While the bread cooks, mash the avocado with the cottage cheese until smooth and creamy.
6. Once the toast is ready, spread the creamy avocado-cottage cheese mix over both slices.
7. Top with a handful of fresh microgreens and optional toppings, if desired.
8. Serve warm, feel the glow, and enjoy your SUPERWELL start to the day.

### WHY IT'S SUPERWELL APPROVED

- ✔ Whole eggs deliver full-spectrum amino acids + choline for brain health.
- ✔ Cottage cheese adds slow-digesting protein and probiotics.
- ✔ Avocado brings healthy fats to stabilize blood sugar and boost skin radiance.
- ✔ Microgreens are rich in antioxidants, phytonutrients, and detoxifying enzymes.

Breakfast Favorites | 65

## SUPERWELL GLOW-UP BAGEL SANDWICH

High-protein, crave-worthy, and ready for your busiest mornings, this SUPERWELL sandwich layers in clean protein, skin-loving fats, and a pop of flavor. It's the perfect balance of nourishment and satisfaction, whether you are on the go or fueling up at home.

**YIELD: 1 SERVING**

- 1 everything bagel, halved and hollowed out
- 2 whole organic eggs
- 1/2 ripe avocado, mashed
- 2 tablespoons organic low-fat Good Culture cottage cheese
- 3 slices of tomato
- 2 tablespoons microgreens (like broccoli or radish sprouts)

### *Optional Toppings*

Everything bagel seasoning, to taste

Drizzle manuka honey (for some sweetness)

Hot sauce (for a spicy kick)

1. Preheat your oven to 375°F and line a baking sheet with parchment.
2. In a small bowl, scramble both eggs until well mixed.
3. Place both hollowed-out bagel halves face up on the baking sheet.
4. Evenly pour the egg mixture into the hollows of both bagel halves.
5. Bake for 12–15 minutes or until eggs are set to your liking.
6. Meanwhile, mash the avocado with the cottage cheese until creamy and spreadable.
7. When the bagels are out of the oven, spread the avocado-cottage cheese mash over one half.
8. Layer with tomato slices and microgreens.
9. Add optional toppings if desired, sandwich it together, and enjoy warm!

### WHY IT'S SUPERWELL APPROVED

✔ Eggs + Cottage Cheese = complete protein to fuel your day

✔ Avocado = skin-loving monounsaturated fats

✔ Microgreens = rich in enzymes, chlorophyll, and antioxidants

✔ Everything Bagel Seasoning = flavorful without extra sauces or sugar

SUPERWELL RECIPES

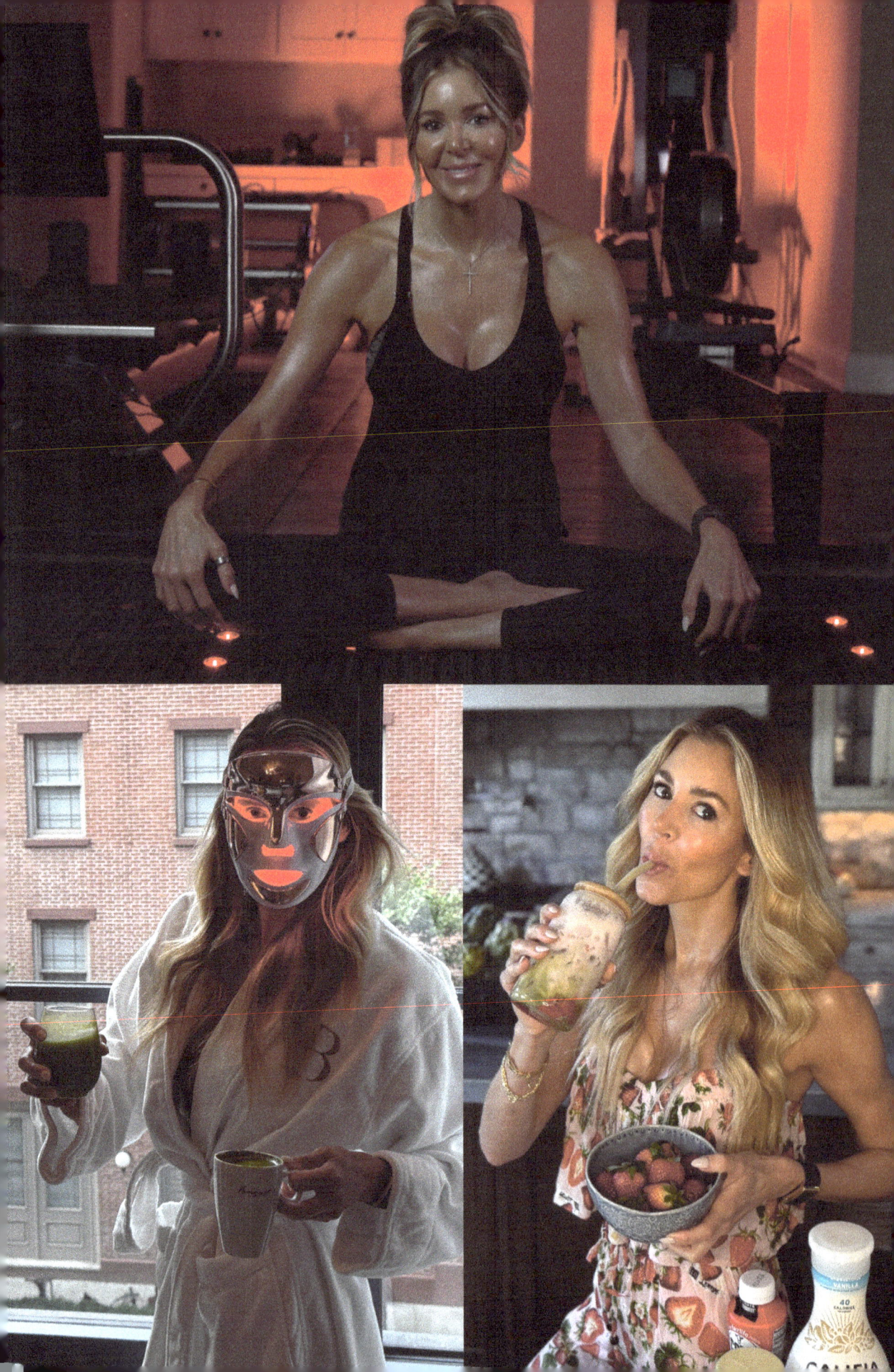

## MULTITASKING WITH INTENTION:
# RED LIGHT, BIOMAT, & MATCHA MORNINGS

One of the most powerful shifts in creating a sustainable morning routine is learning how to *layer* your wellness practices with purpose. I start each day by slipping on my red light therapy mask: a simple, effective way to stimulate collagen, reduce inflammation, and support cellular regeneration while I move through my early morning rituals. While the red light does its work, I'm setting intentions for the day, heating up my BioMat (more on that in a bit), feeding my dogs, and prepping my signature SUPERWELL matcha.

Once those quiet tasks are complete, the mask comes off and the next phase begins: I settle onto the warmed BioMat and soak in the infrared heat while sipping my matcha, letting the grounding warmth activate circulation, support detoxification, and ease my body into a state of focused calm.

This is how I build momentum through science-backed practices done with ease and intention. These moments aren't just multitasking; they are a blueprint for starting the day in alignment with energy, presence, and purpose.

# BIOMAT BRILLIANCE

## HARNESSING INFRARED HEAT FOR CELLULAR VITALITY

One of the first things I do each morning before stepping outside for morning sun and grounding is turn on my BioMat to begin heating up while I habit stack with other SUPERWELL practices. This medical device uses far infrared (FIR) heat, negative ions, and amethyst crystals to penetrate heat deep into tissues, promoting cellular detoxification, improved circulation, and nervous system regulation. FIR therapy has been shown to enhance mitochondrial function, boost nitric oxide production for vascular health, and reduce systemic inflammation: all crucial for longevity and overall vitality. As I sit on the BioMat, I allow its therapeutic warmth to stimulate blood flow, relax tense muscles, and prime my body for optimal recovery. Research indicates that FIR therapy activates heat shock proteins, which aid in cellular repair and resilience, reinforcing why this has become a cornerstone of my morning routine.

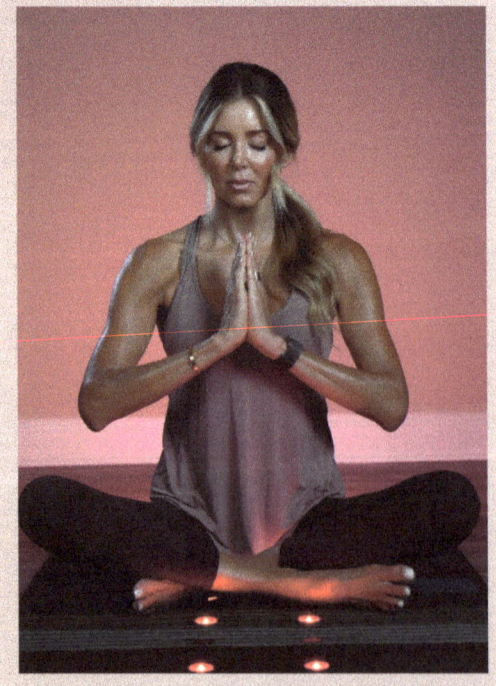

This deep-penetrating heat doesn't just provide relaxation; it kickstarts my lymphatic system, accelerates detoxification, and enhances parasympathetic nervous system activation. By incorporating the BioMat into my habit-stacking ritual, I set the foundation for a calm yet energized state, priming my body for my upcoming infrared sauna session, allowing for an even greater internal heat activation and compounding the benefits of thermotherapy. Studies show that consistent FIR exposure can improve sleep quality, enhance immune function, and even support metabolic health by mimicking the effects of moderate exercise. For me, this isn't just a wellness tool; it's an integral part of my longevity strategy, ensuring that each day begins with cellular regeneration, nervous system balance, and optimized energy levels.

## RELAXATION

The BioMat promotes deep relaxation using advanced infrared pulsed electromagnetic field (PEMF) technology. By harnessing the power of FIR light and pulsed electromagnetic fields, it helps soothe muscles, reduce stress, and promote a profound sense of calm. This innovative technology works to enhance overall wellbeing by supporting relaxation and recovery at a deep level.

## PAIN RELIEF

The BioMat effectively reduces pain and inflammation by improving blood circulation. Its advanced FIR and PEMF technology stimulates blood flow, which helps deliver more oxygen and nutrients to affected areas while removing toxins. This enhanced circulation supports the body's natural healing processes, alleviating discomfort and reducing inflammation for a more comfortable and balanced state of wellbeing.

## ENHANCED MOOD

Regular use of the BioMat can elevate your mood by alleviating stress and anxiety. The combination of FIR and PEMF technology promotes relaxation and helps regulate stress levels, leading to a more balanced and positive emotional state. This consistent use supports mental wellbeing, contributing to an overall sense of calm and improved mood.

## IMPROVED SLEEP

The relaxation benefits of the BioMat also extend to improved sleep quality. By reducing stress and soothing muscles, it helps create a more restful environment for sleep, leading to deeper, more restorative rest. This enhanced relaxation contributes to a more consistent and rejuvenating sleep experience, supporting overall wellbeing.

## HEALING BENEFITS

The BioMat supports overall healing and wellbeing by providing a spa-like experience right in your office. Its advanced technology promotes relaxation, alleviates stress, and enhances comfort, creating a soothing environment that fosters both physical and mental rejuvenation. This combination of benefits helps you maintain a balanced and refreshed state, even during busy workdays.

# MATCHA MASTERY

## A SMARTER ENERGY SOLUTION FOR MIND & BODY

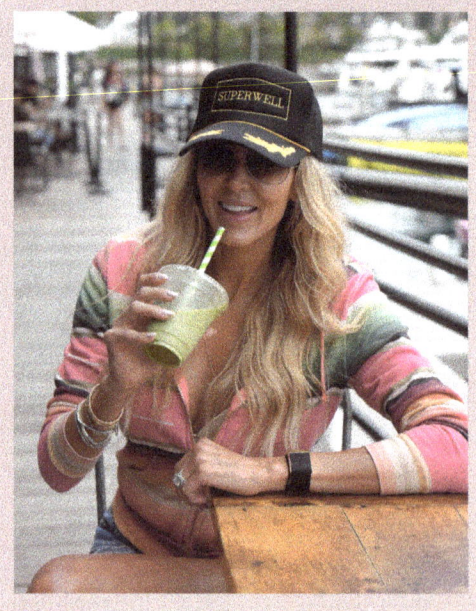

Switching from coffee to matcha has been one of the most impactful upgrades to my morning routine, transforming the way I fuel my body and mind. Unlike coffee, which can trigger cortisol spikes, blood sugar fluctuations, and energy crashes, matcha provides a steady, sustained release of energy due to its unique combination of L-theanine and naturally occurring caffeine.

L-theanine, an amino acid found in matcha, promotes alpha brain waves, which enhance focus, mental clarity, and relaxation without the jitters or anxiety associated with traditional caffeine sources. Studies show that matcha can increase thermogenesis (calorie burning) by up to 40%, support metabolic function, and provide a potent dose of catechins, which are powerful antioxidants that combat oxidative stress, support liver detoxification, and enhance cognitive function.

To further optimize this ritual, I add 5 grams of creatine to my morning matcha, a powerhouse supplement known for enhancing adenosine triphosphate (ATP) production, supporting brain health, and increasing muscle performance and recovery. This small but strategic shift was guided by real-time data from my WHOOP and Levels health app continuous glucose monitor (CGM), confirming that matcha helps regulate glucose levels, supports metabolic flexibility, and provides long-lasting energy without the crash.

**Pro Tip:** Want to amplify the benefits even more? Froth in a scoop of unsweetened vanilla protein powder to create a *super*-charged matcha that supports your protein intake from the moment your day begins. Prioritizing protein early in the day has been shown to improve satiety, stabilize blood sugar, support lean muscle maintenance, and kickstart your metabolism. This is a delicious, functional way to front-load your nutrition without compromise.

This intentional morning ritual is more than a drink; it's a blueprint-aligned habit that supports sustainable energy, sharper cognition, and metabolic resilience. Welcome to the smarter, calmer, more empowered way to start your day—SUPERWELL style!

## COGNITIVE FUNCTION

Adding creatine to your matcha tea can boost brain function and focus. Creatine, known for its cognitive benefits, complements the mental clarity provided by matcha tea's natural compounds. This combination enhances cognitive performance, helping you stay sharp and focused throughout the day.

## MUSCLE GROWTH

Creatine supports muscle growth and aids in recovery after workouts. By increasing the availability of energy in muscle cells, it enhances performance during exercise and accelerates the repair and rebuilding of muscle tissue, leading to more effective training and faster recovery.

## PHYSICAL PERFORMANCE

This supplement enhances overall physical performance and endurance. By improving energy levels and optimizing muscle function, it supports more effective workouts and prolonged physical activity, helping you achieve better results and sustain peak performance.

## METABOLISM BOOST

Matcha boosts metabolism, which aids in weight management. By enhancing your body's ability to burn calories more efficiently, it supports your weight loss goals and helps maintain a healthy weight.

## ANTIOXIDANTS

Matcha is packed with antioxidants that promote overall health and wellbeing, offering a steady stream of energy throughout the day. Its unique combination of nutrients supports a vibrant lifestyle while avoiding the jittery side effects often associated with coffee. By enhancing your energy levels and providing a more stable boost, matcha helps you stay focused and alert without the usual coffee crashes.

# SUPERWELL
# Simple Matcha

*A morning ritual designed to energize, balance, and nourish without the crash.*

Matcha is my daily go-to for calm, focused energy. Unlike coffee, matcha provides a steady lift thanks to its natural pairing of L-theanine and slow-releasing caffeine. This latte supports mental clarity, metabolic health, and glowing skin—all while tasting delicious. And if you want to supercharge your routine? Add a scoop of clean protein and creatine to make it a powerhouse for the brain and body. This is not just a matcha latte—it's your SUPERWELL moment. One small ritual. One intentional shift. One powerful way to start your day in alignment.

- 1 cup unsweetened vanilla almond milk or milk of choice
- 1 teaspoon high-quality matcha powder (ceremonial-grade preferred), to taste
- 1–2 tablespoons filtered water
- 1 tablespoon pure maple syrup, or to taste
- Dash of Ceylon cinnamon
- Ice (for iced version)

## Optional Add-Ins

- 1/2 cup (1 scoop) unsweetened vanilla protein powder (for muscle support and satiety)
- 5 g creatine monohydrate (for strength, focus, and cellular energy)
- 1 teaspoon collagen peptides powder or MCT oil (for glowing skin and metabolic fuel)

## HOT MATCHA LATTE

1. Warm your almond milk in a small saucepan until it reaches 150–160°F—steamy but not boiling—to preserve antioxidants and nutrients.

2. In a separate mug, whisk matcha powder with 1 tablespoon of hot (~175°F) water until smooth and frothy.

3. Stir in maple syrup, cinnamon, and your desired SUPERWELL add-ins. Froth or blend to combine.

4. Slowly pour warm milk into your matcha mixture while stirring. Use a frother for a creamy finish.

5. Sit, sip, and let your nervous system ease into the day.

## ICED MATCHA LATTE

1. In a shaker or glass, combine matcha powder with 2 tablespoons of room-temperature water. Whisk until smooth.

2. Stir in maple syrup and your preferred SUPERWELL add-ins, like protein and creatine.

3. Add cold almond milk, stir gently, then pour over a glass of ice.

4. Sprinkle with cinnamon or add a spoonful of cold foam (see note) on top if desired.

### PRO TIPS

For a cold foam topper, blend 1/4 cup cold almond milk with a touch of vanilla protein powder and froth until thick. Spoon over your iced matcha for an indulgent yet functional finish.

My favorite go-to matcha brands are Matcha Made Latte Grande and Chamberlain Coffee Vanilla Matcha.

"WELL" IS WHERE YOU BEGIN.
*Superwell is where you belong.*

SUPERWELL RECIPES

## Strawberry
# MATCHA GLOW SWIRL

This refreshing fusion of antioxidant-rich strawberries and calming, energizing matcha is layered for beauty and built for function. Subtly sweet, this protein-optional drink is more than just a pretty swirl. It supports sustained energy, stable blood sugar, and glowing skin—a delicious, nourishing way to start (or brighten) your day.

**YIELD: 1 SERVING**

### WHY IT'S SUPERWELL APPROVED

✓ Zen Basil seeds = fiber, omegas, potassium + glow from within

✓ Matcha = calm energy, antioxidants, skin support

✓ Strawberries = vitamin C for collagen and radiance

✓ Protein options = blood sugar balance + satiety

---

1 cup organic frozen strawberries, thawed, or 6–8 fresh strawberries, some juice reserved

1 tablespoon Zen Basil seeds, soaked overnight in 1/4 cup water (optional)

1–2 cups small, round, pebble-style ice (use silicone ball molds for best effect)

**MILK LAYER (CHOOSE ONE):**
1-1/2 cups Core Power Strawberry Protein Shake (26 g protein)

1-1/2 cups unsweetened almond milk + 1/2 cup (1 scoop) berry protein powder of choice (30 g protein)

1-1/2 cups unsweetened almond milk or milk of choice (no added protein)

**MATCHA LAYER:**
1 teaspoon high-quality matcha powder, to taste (see note)

2–3 tablespoons hot (not boiling) water

**STRAWBERRY VANILLA COLD FOAM:**
1/4 cup Chobani Vanilla Coffee Creamer (or clean alternative)

1–2 teaspoons leftover muddled strawberry juice

**GARNISH (OPTIONAL):**
Strawberry slice
Mint sprig
Matcha dust

---

1. Spoon the muddled strawberries into the bottom of your glass.
2. Add soaked Zen Basil seeds, if using, for that fiber-rich, omega-3 boost.
3. Add pebble ice until your glass is three-quarters full.
4. Pour in your milk layer of choice.
5. Whisk your matcha paste until smooth and frothy, then swirl it over the milk layer.
6. Froth together the creamer and strawberry juice with a milk frother until fluffy. Top the Strawberry Matcha Glow Swirl with your strawberry vanilla cold foam.
7. Optional: Garnish with a strawberry slice, mint sprig, or matcha dust.

# Superwell Protein
## POWER MATCHA

*High-vibe. Protein-fueled. Creatine-enhanced. Anti-inflammatory.*

It's not just matcha—it's your daily ritual for strength, glow, and grace.

- 1 heaping teaspoon organic matcha powder (I sometimes use 2 teaspoons for an extra kick!)
- 1–2 tablespoons hot water (160–175°F—not boiling to protect antioxidants)
- 1 cup unsweetened vanilla almond milk
- 1/2 cup (1 scoop) VEGA French Vanilla Protein Powder
- 3–5 grams (1 scoop) THORNE Creatine
- Pebble ice

**OPTIONAL ADD-INS**
- 1/4 cup Chobani Vanilla Coffee Creamer + 1 teaspoon almond milk
- Cinnamon for topping

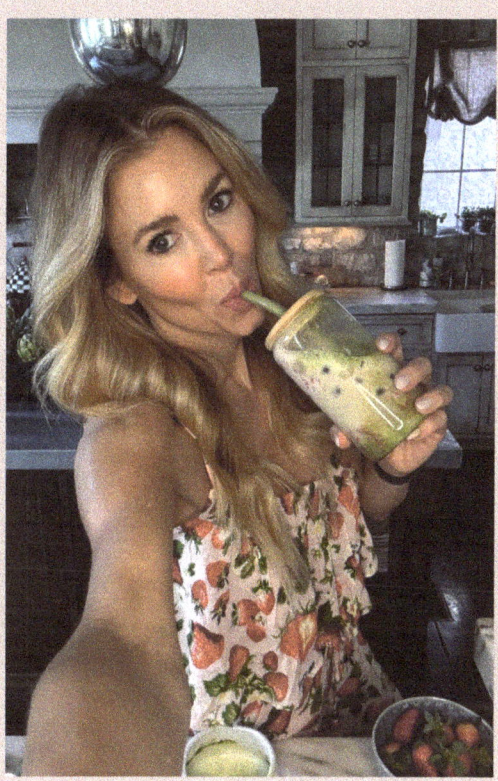

1. In a matcha bowl, whisk matcha powder with hot water until smooth, fluffy, and vibrant.
2. In a separate mug or frother, combine almond milk, protein, and creatine. Froth or whisk until creamy.
3. Fill a cute glass (I like Tang Pin's aesthetic matcha glass) with pebble ice. Pour in your almond milk blend. Re-whisk your matcha paste and swirl it on top for that signature green cascade.
4. To make the optional cloud topping, froth the coffee creamer with a splash of leftover almond milk. Pour on top and sprinkle with cinnamon.

### WHY IT'S SUPERWELL APPROVED

✔ Protein = muscle + skin repair

✔ Creatine = strength + cognitive clarity

✔ Matcha = gentle energy + antioxidants

✔ Cinnamon = anti-inflammatory bonus

# GLOW RITUALS

## AS NERVOUS SYSTEM NOURISHMENT

Skincare is more than a beauty routine. It is a sacred window of self-connection. When approached intentionally, it becomes a practice of nervous system nourishment, energetic recalibration, and cellular-level renewal. I no longer view skincare as a "to-do"; it is a sanctuary. A moment to reconnect, to slow down, and to anchor myself in the now.

Start by creating an atmosphere that speaks to your senses. Light a candle. Play soft, grounding music. Dim the lights. Let the environment invite your body to exhale. Then begin your ritual with presence.

### THE POWER OF LYMPHATIC FLOW

One of the most overlooked yet essential keys to glowing skin is lymphatic drainage. Your lymphatic system helps eliminate toxins, regulate fluids, and support immune health, but unlike your circulatory system, it has no built-in pump. It depends on your movement, breath, and gentle stimulation.

Lymphatic facial massage supports this natural detoxification. Just a few minutes of upward, outward strokes using your fingertips, a chilled gua sha tool, or a facial wand can de-puff, stimulate circulation, and bring your skin back to life. Always begin at the neck to open the drainage pathways, then work upward across the jawline, cheeks, and forehead. Think of it as your glow after flow.

### HYDRATION AND BARRIER REPAIR

Hydration is a non-negotiable when it comes to youthful, radiant skin. Well-hydrated skin maintains its natural barrier, which protects against environmental stressors, reduces sensitivity, and prevents premature aging. As the seasons change, so should your hydration strategy. In warmer months, focus on replenishing fluids lost through heat and sweat. In colder months, combat dryness from indoor heating with richer creams, facial oils, and hydrating masks.

Seal your ritual with antioxidant-packed oils or balms that strengthen the skin barrier, reduce inflammation, and boost elasticity. The goal is to nourish, not strip; to replenish, not chase perfection.

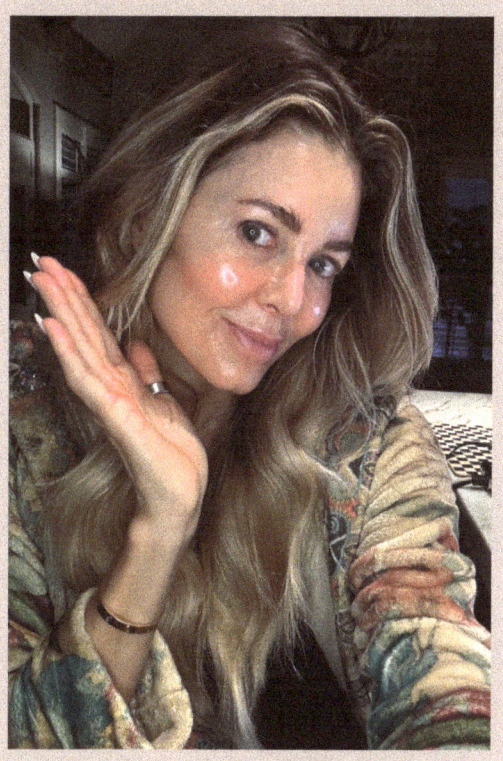

## SUPERWELL SKINCARE IN PRACTICE

Each day, I treat my skincare time as an extension of my wellness practice. I often layer in deep breathing—inhale for four, hold for four, exhale for six; or repeat grounding mantras to calm my mind as I massage in each product. This stacks the benefits: It regulates cortisol, activates your parasympathetic nervous system, and prepares you for deeper sleep.

These are not vanity habits. These are foundational practices in nervous system regulation, lymphatic flow, and self-respect. When done with intention, your skin reflects more than a glow—it reflects a state of peace.

### SUPERWELL TIP

You don't need dozens of steps to achieve results. Consistency and presence matter more than perfection. Pair this time with breathwork, soft music, or silence. Let your skincare become your sanctuary.

When you support your inner landscape, your outer glow follows. That is the SUPERWELL approach to skincare: intuitive, restorative, and rooted in love.

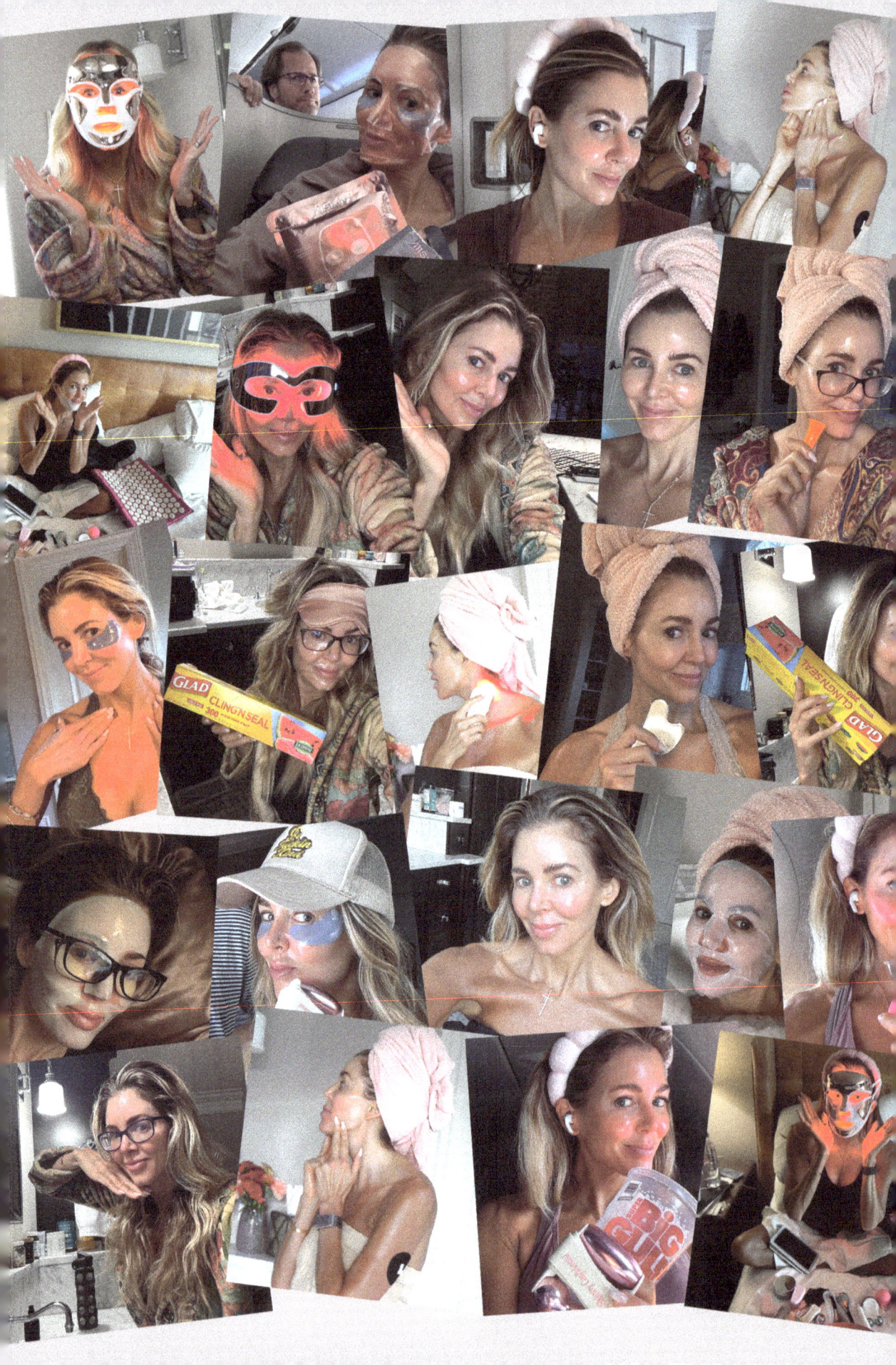

A.M. GLASS

# SKIN ROUTINE

### 1. CLEANSE: MAY LINDSTROM'S THE PENDULUM POTION

- A luxurious, antioxidant-rich cleansing oil that melts away impurities while protecting the skin's natural barrier.
- Contains a nourishing blend of camellia, avocado, and cacao oils to balance and soften the skin.
- Use a gentle lymphatic drainage massage to wake up the skin, reduce puffiness, and boost circulation.

### 2. DRY: CLEAN SKIN CLUB CLEAN TOWELS XL

- Single-use, biodegradable, ultra-soft towels that prevent reintroducing bacteria to freshly cleansed skin
- Gentle and hygienic—perfect for sensitive or acne-prone skin

### 3. LED THERAPY: DR. DENNIS GROSS DRX SPECTRALITE FACEWARE PRO LED MASK

- Red light stimulates collagen and elastin, reducing fine lines, wrinkles, and loss of firmness.
- Blue light fights acne-causing bacteria, calms inflammation, and prevents breakouts.
- Why I love it: I wear it while multitasking—making matcha, grounding outside, or playing with the dogs.

## 3. CRYO DE-PUFFING: 111SKIN CRYO DE-PUFFING EYE MASKS

- Cooling masks reduce puffiness, dark circles, and fatigue around the eyes.
- Hydrating hydrogel formula helps brighten, calm, and plump the delicate eye area.

## 4. MIST BETWEEN LAYERS: EMINENCE ORGANIC STONE CROP HYDRATING MIST

- Deeply hydrates, brightens, and calms the skin with stone crop.
- Boosts absorption of products layered afterward.
- Seals in hydration for maximum results.

**Pro Tip:** Use as the "glue" for a lit-from-within look.

## 5. BRIGHTEN & FIRM: DR. DENNIS GROSS VITAMIN C LACTIC 15% SERUM

- Brightens skin tone, evens discoloration, and stimulates collagen production with vitamin C and lactic acid.

**Pro Tip:** Lactic acid exfoliates gently, allowing vitamin C to penetrate deeper for maximum glow.

## 6. GROWTH FACTOR BOOST: SKINMEDICA TNS ADVANCED+ GROWTH FACTOR SERUM

- Accelerates skin repair, improves texture, and reduces deep lines and wrinkles.
- I call it "Botox in a bottle."
- Boosts collagen production and enhances skin elasticity.
- Worth it: A little goes a long way, with transformative results over time.

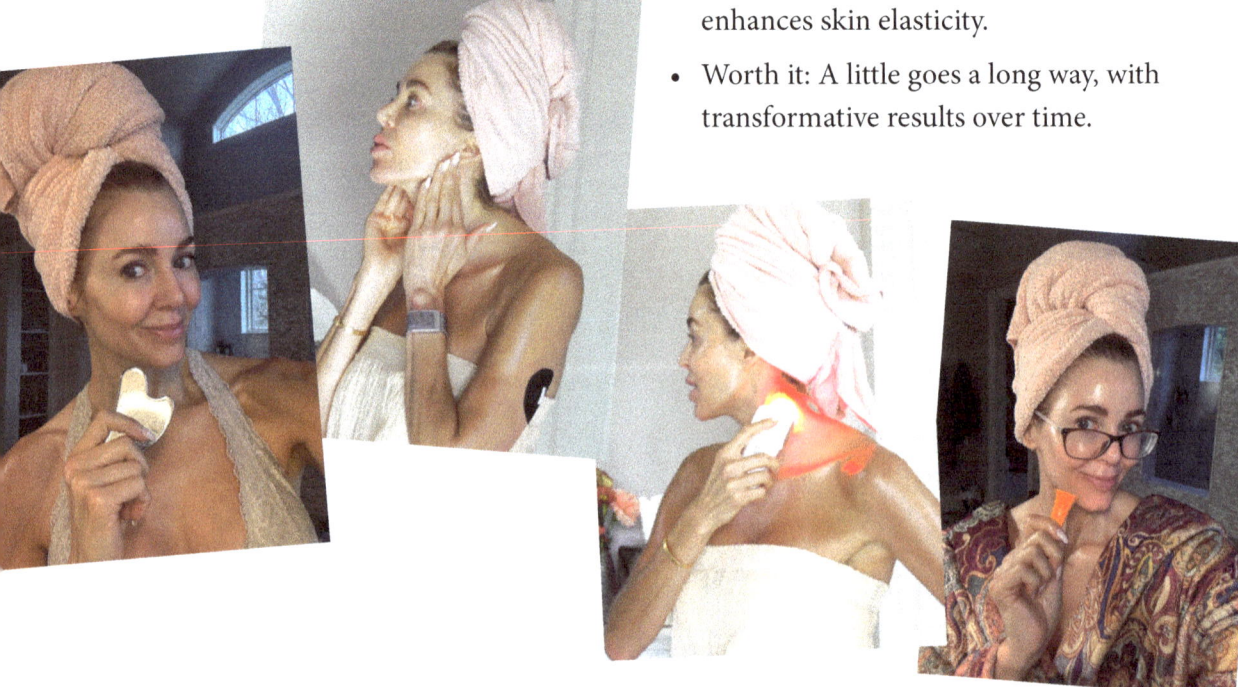

## 7. HYDRATION POWER DUO: SKINCEUTICALS HYDRATING B5 GEL + HYALURONIC ACID INTENSIFIER

- Hydrating B5 gel: Lightweight serum with vitamin B5 and hyaluronic acid to replenish moisture.
- Hyaluronic acid intensifier: Enhances hyaluronic acid levels, improving hydration and elasticity.
- Why I mix them: This duo creates a hydration cocktail for bouncy, supple skin, especially in colder months.

## 8. NOURISH: LE PRUNIER BEAUTY OIL

- Organic plum seed oil is rich in antioxidants, soothes inflammation, balances moisture, and protects against environmental damage.
- Smells as good as it feels—like almond butter cookies—pure, natural, and heavenly!

## 9. EYE PERFECTION: SISLEY PARIS EYE CONTOUR MASK

- Ultra-hydrating eye mask reduces fine lines, de-puffs, and keeps the under-eye area smooth and dewy.
- Keeps dryness and crepiness at bay for a youthful, refreshed look.

## 10. SEAL & HYDRATE: U BEAUTY THE SUPER HYDRATOR

- Silky moisturizer with hydration-boosting siren capsules targets dry areas, smoothes fine lines, and improves elasticity.
- Why I love it: It gives your skin that perfect, plump finish.

## 11. SPF PROTECTION + GLOW: COLORESCIENCE SUNFORGETTABLE TOTAL PROTECTION FACE SHIELD FLEX SPF 50 (MEDIUM)

- Lightweight, tinted SPF with broad-spectrum protection that adapts to your skin tone.
- Leaves a beautiful, silky glow without greasiness.

## 12. FINAL TOUCH FOR EXTRA GLOW: MONASTERY ATTAR FLORAL REPAIR CONCENTRATE

- Rich, reparative balm with botanicals to nourish and soften.
- Dab onto high points—forehead, cheeks, nose—for extra glass-skin radiance.

# CONTRAST THERAPY:

## MASTERING THE ELEMENTS

### Harnessing Heat & Cold for Peak Performance

Contrast therapy is a powerful practice of alternating between intense heat and cold exposure. It is a scientifically backed method to enhance resilience, recovery, and metabolic efficiency. This deliberate exposure to extreme temperatures trains your body to adapt to stress, fortifies the immune system, and improves cardiovascular function. The heat phase dilates blood vessels, increases circulation, and deeply relaxes muscles, while the cold phase constricts blood vessels, reduces inflammation, and activates brown fat for metabolic enhancement. More than just physical benefits, contrast therapy serves as a training ground for the nervous system, teaching the body how to shift between stress and relaxation with greater ease. The ability to control these responses is a key component of SUPERWELL Living—building resilience not only in the body but also in the mind.

### CIRCULATION & CARDIOVASCULAR OPTIMIZATION

The rapid expansion and constriction of blood vessels caused by contrast therapy strengthens the vascular system, much like a workout for your cardiovascular health. Heat exposure improves blood flow, oxygen delivery, and nutrient transport to tissues, while cold exposure reduces inflammation and enhances vasoconstriction, preventing blood pooling and improving overall circulation efficiency. Regular contrast therapy has been shown to improve endothelial function, reduce blood pressure, and support heart health over time.

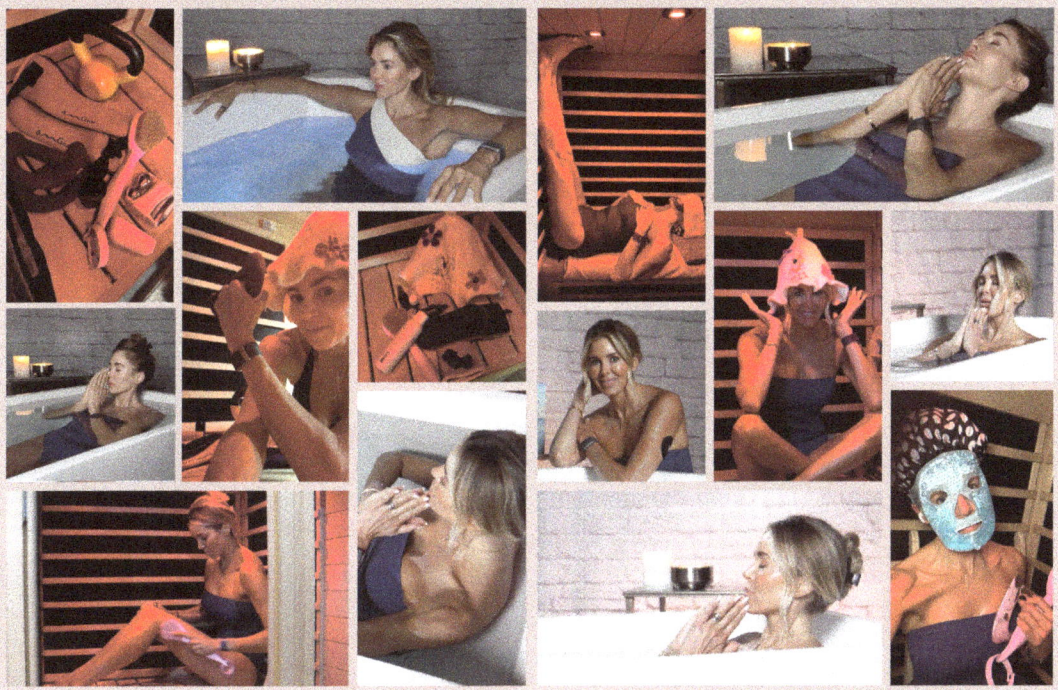

## RECOVERY & MUSCLE REGENERATION

By alternating between vasodilation (heat) and vasoconstriction (cold), contrast therapy flushes metabolic waste from muscles, accelerates tissue repair, and reduces post-exercise soreness. Heat therapy relaxes muscles, enhances flexibility, and improves nutrient delivery, while cold therapy reduces inflammation, numbs pain receptors, and prevents excessive swelling. This combination makes contrast therapy one of the most effective natural recovery tools for athletes and active individuals.

## IMMUNE SYSTEM FORTIFICATION

The deliberate stress introduced by heat and cold exposure stimulates the production of heat shock proteins (HSPs) and cold shock proteins (CSPs), both of which play crucial roles in cellular repair, immune defense, and longevity. Heat therapy increases white blood cell production, enhancing immune surveillance, while cold exposure activates brown fat, supporting metabolic function and improving resilience to illness. This hormetic stressor trains the body to respond more efficiently to environmental changes, reducing susceptibility to infections and inflammatory diseases.

## METABOLIC & ENERGY BOOST

Cold exposure activates brown adipose tissue (BAT), a metabolically active type of fat that burns calories to generate heat. This process, known as non-shivering thermogenesis, helps increase calorie expenditure, regulate blood sugar levels, and support insulin sensitivity. Heat exposure further enhances mitochondrial function, improving energy production and metabolic efficiency. By incorporating contrast therapy, you train your body to become more metabolically flexible, enhancing endurance, fat-burning potential, and sustained energy levels.

### HOW TO PRACTICE 4-7-8 BREATHWORK

1. **Find a Comfortable Position.** Whether you are seated or lying down, make sure you are in a comfortable position where you can fully relax.

2. **Place the Tip of Your Tongue.** Lightly touch the roof of your mouth with the tip of your tongue, just behind your front teeth.

3. **Inhale Through Your Nose (4 Seconds).** Close your mouth and inhale quietly through your nose to a count of 4, drawing the breath deeply into your diaphragm and belly—expanding fully and allowing your body to take in oxygen where it's most nourishing.

4. **Hold Your Breath (7 Seconds).** Hold your breath for a count of 7. Stay calm and relaxed.

5. **Exhale Through Your Mouth (8 Seconds).** Exhale completely through your mouth, making a whooshing sound, to a count of 8.

6. **Repeat the Cycle.** Repeat this cycle for 4 rounds initially. Over time, you can increase to 8 cycles as you feel more comfortable.

#### Pro Tips:

- Use this technique twice daily for the best results.
- It's a powerful tool for calming the nervous system, aiding sleep, and reducing anxiety.

## PARASYMPATHETIC MASTERY: CONTROLLING THE NERVOUS SYSTEM

Contrast therapy is a powerful tool for training the autonomic nervous system, allowing you to intentionally shift between stress states. Cold exposure initially activates the sympathetic nervous system (fight-or-flight response), spiking norepinephrine, increasing alertness, and stimulating circulation. However, through breathwork and intentional relaxation, you can override this response, activating the parasympathetic nervous system (rest-and-digest state). This teaches the body how to transition from high-stress states into deep relaxation more efficiently, strengthening overall nervous system resilience. Meditation, breath control, and gradual adaptation to cold immersion can enhance vagal tone, reduce stress hormone production, and create a lasting sense of calm even in life's most intense moments.

Contrast therapy is more than just heat and cold; it's a form of physiological training that enhances mental fortitude, stress resilience, and total-body recovery. By making these intentional shifts daily, you are not just adapting to stress . . . you are mastering it!

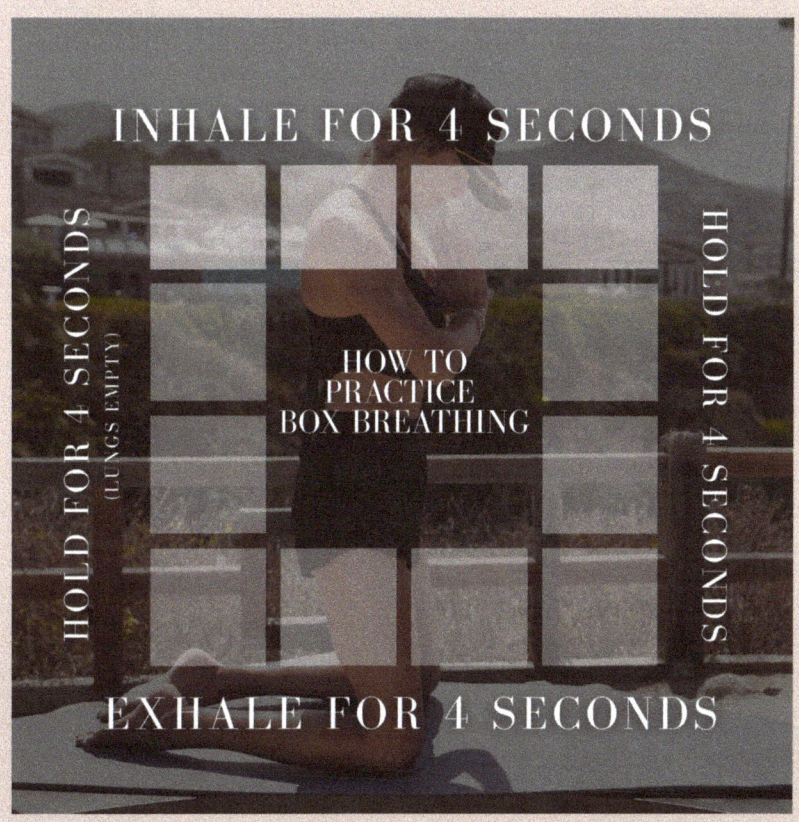

# SAUNA SANCTUARY:

## THE SCIENCE OF HEAT FOR DETOX, LONGEVITY, & DEEP RESTORATION

Infrared and traditional saunas have long been recognized for their powerful physiological benefits, extending far beyond relaxation. Heat therapy stimulates circulation, enhances cardiovascular function, activates heat shock proteins (HSPs), and promotes cellular resilience. Research shows that consistent sauna use can reduce the risk of cardiovascular disease by up to 50%, improve mitochondrial function, and enhance detoxification by increasing sweat-induced elimination of heavy metals like mercury, lead, and cadmium. Regular sauna exposure has also been linked to a 40% decrease in all-cause mortality due to its impact on heart health, inflammation reduction, and neuroprotection. For me, sauna sessions are not just about sweating. It is a deeply restorative, intentional practice that helps me recalibrate my nervous system, optimize recovery, and elevate my overall wellbeing.

To transform each sauna session into a SUPERWELL ritual, I begin with dry brushing, a practice that stimulates lymphatic drainage, enhances circulation, and primes the skin for detoxification. This preparatory step boosts the sauna's ability to flush out toxins and promote deeper sweat-induced cleansing. I also incorporate facial sculpting techniques to encourage lymphatic movement and support a youthful, oxygenated complexion. As the heat gradually builds, I immerse myself in meditation, a scientifically backed technique shown to reduce cortisol, lower blood pressure, and enhance parasympathetic activation for deep relaxation. This layered approach amplifies the sauna's effects, allowing me to maximize its metabolic, neurological, and cardiovascular benefits. By combining heat therapy with intentional recovery strategies, I create an integrated wellness practice that rejuvenates both body and mind, ensuring that each session leaves me feeling deeply restored, energized, and primed for optimal health.

## DETOXIFICATION

Sauna sessions promote detoxification by encouraging sweating, which helps the body expel toxins. As you sweat, your skin releases impurities and waste products, supporting the body's natural cleansing processes and leaving you feeling refreshed and rejuvenated.

## SKIN HEALTH

Increased blood flow enhances skin health and appearance by delivering more oxygen and nutrients to skin cells. This improved circulation helps to rejuvenate the skin, boost its natural glow, and promote a more youthful and radiant complexion.

## STRESS RELIEF

The heat relaxes muscles and alleviates stress by soothing tightness and promoting a sense of calm. This warmth helps ease muscle tension and creates an environment conducive to relaxation and overall wellbeing.

## IMPROVED CIRCULATION

Enhanced circulation supports cardiovascular health by improving blood flow and reducing strain on the heart. This increased circulation helps to deliver oxygen and nutrients more efficiently, while also aiding in the removal of waste products from the bloodstream, contributing to overall heart health and wellness.

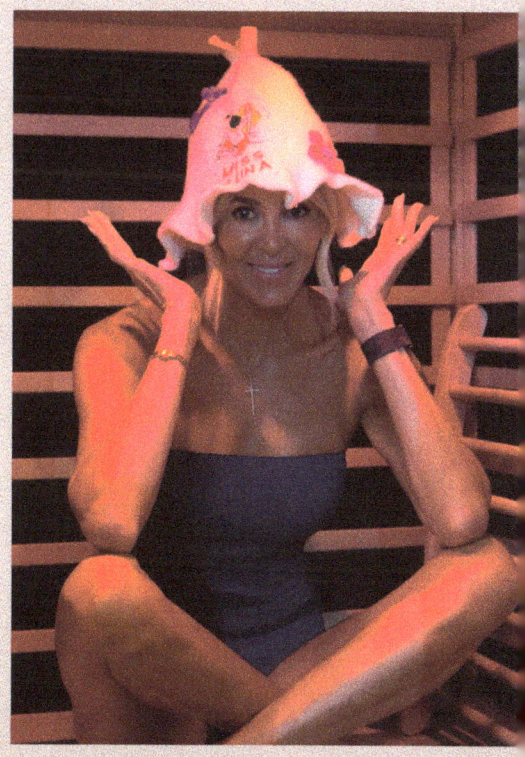

## IMMUNE BOOST

Regular sauna use strengthens the immune system by stimulating the production of white blood cells and improving overall circulation. This enhanced immune response helps the body better defend against infections and supports overall health and resilience.

# SWEAT, STACK, & SAVOR:
# HABIT STACKING FOR THE ULTIMATE SAUNA RITUAL

If you think a sauna session is just sitting and sweating, think again—this is prime time to layer in high-impact wellness practices and truly elevate your mind, body, and spirit. I make every minute inside my sauna count by habit-stacking multiple SUPERWELL practices, customizing each session based on what my body is craving that day. Some days, it's a deep reset with breathwork and meditation, and other days, I'm breaking a sweat while sculpting my arms with light weights. The key? Keep it fun, intentional, and something you look forward to!

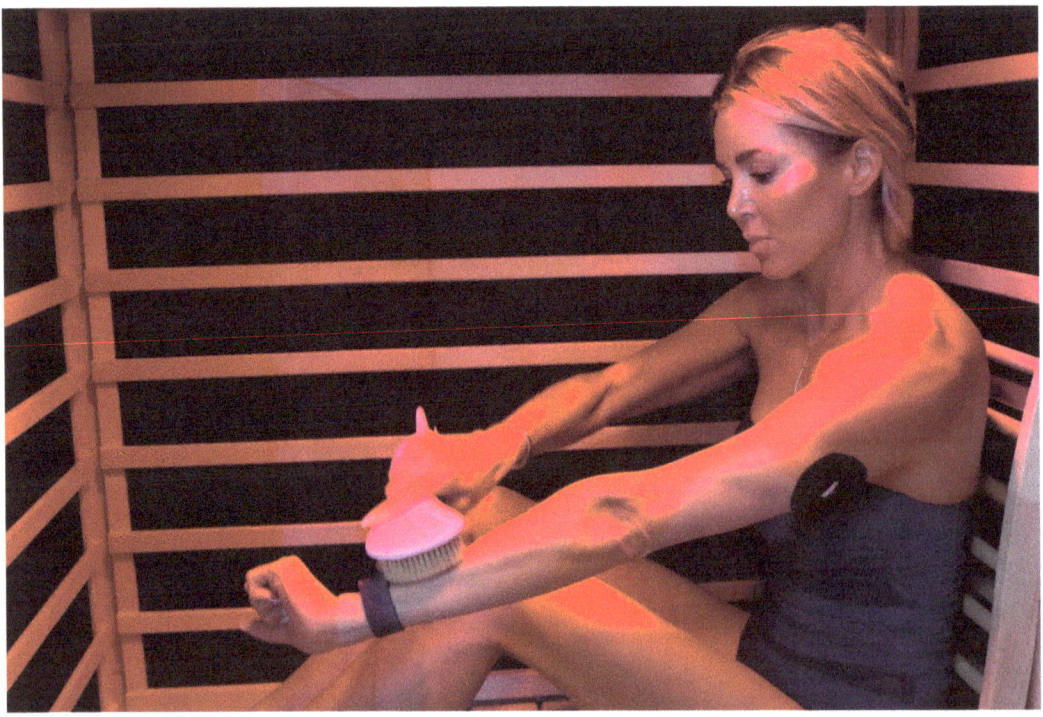

## HOW I MAXIMIZE MY SAUNA SESSIONS

- **Red Light Therapy** – Always on for collagen production, cellular repair, and muscle recovery.
- **Dry Brushing** – Stimulates lymphatic drainage, exfoliates skin, and kickstarts circulation.
- **Ice Roller for Facial Sculpting & Depuffing** – Nothing like a hot/cold contrast to wake up the skin and boost circulation.
- **20-Minute Meditation** – Meditation or guided breathwork decreases stress, improves focus, and shifts into full relaxation mode
- **Aromatherapy** – I use essential oils to set the tone, whether I need energy or deep relaxation.
  - For an Energizing Boost – Try peppermint, eucalyptus, or rosemary—all known to stimulate the senses, enhance focus, and promote mental clarity.
  - For Calming & Grounding – Use lavender, chamomile, or frankincense to soothe the nervous system, deepen relaxation, and support emotional balance.
- **Listen & Learn** – This is a great time to tune into a podcast, catch up on an audiobook, or even call a friend for a heart-to-heart.
- **Journaling & Intention Setting** – The heat opens the mind as much as it opens the pores—perfect for reflecting, goal setting, or simply jotting down thoughts.
- **Mini Sauna Workout** – A light 20-minute arm toning routine is my go-to—because why not get a sculpting session in while I sweat?
- **Silence & Stillness** – Sometimes, I ditch all the stimulation and just sit in total silence—because in a world of constant noise, the quiet can be the most powerful reset.

Every sauna session is a choose-your-own-adventure experience . . . some days, I focus on deep relaxation, and other days, I lean into high-performance recovery. This sacred time is completely customizable to what my mind, body, and spirit are asking for. By making it intentional and enjoyable, sauna time becomes less of a "wellness to-do" and more of a ritual I can't wait to step into.

# WHAT ARE THE BENEFITS OF
# DRY BRUSHING?

### STIMULATES LYMPHATIC FLOW AND DETOXIFICATION

Dry brushing encourages the movement of lymph fluid through the lymphatic system, which is essential for removing toxins, waste, and pathogens from the body. This process supports immune health and helps maintain a balanced internal environment.

### EXFOLIATES DEAD SKIN CELLS

The gentle bristles of a dry brush effectively remove dead skin cells, promoting cell turnover and leaving the skin smoother and more vibrant. This also enhances the absorption of skincare products for improved hydration and nourishment.

### BOOSTS CIRCULATION

Dry brushing improves blood flow to the skin's surface, delivering oxygen and essential nutrients to the tissues. This increased circulation promotes a healthy glow and supports overall skin vitality.

### SUPPORTS HORMONAL AND DIGESTIVE HEALTH

By activating the nervous system and improving lymph and blood flow, dry brushing indirectly supports hormonal balance and digestive processes, aiding in the body's natural regulatory functions.

### ENERGIZES THE BODY AND MIND

The invigorating nature of dry brushing not only stimulates the skin but also provides a refreshing boost of energy. Many find it helps improve focus and mental clarity by reducing stress and promoting a sense of wellbeing.

## CREATIVE WAYS TO EXPERIENCE
# HEAT SHOCK THERAPY
*(No Fancy Sauna Needed!)*

Heat shock therapy isn't just for those with high-end infrared saunas—you can still harness the power of heat exposure using accessible, budget-friendly methods. Whether you are looking for deep relaxation, detoxification, muscle recovery, or metabolic benefits, here are 10 creative ways to incorporate heat shock therapy into your wellness routine without an expensive sauna setup.

### 1. HOT SHOWERS WITH STEAM BOOST

- Turn your shower as hot as you can tolerate and let the steam build up.
- Stay in for 10–15 minutes, focusing on deep breathing to increase circulation and relaxation.
- To intensify the detox, add essential oils like eucalyptus, peppermint, or tea tree for respiratory benefits.

## 2. DIY STEAM ROOM IN YOUR BATHROOM

- Run hot water in the shower with the door closed to create a steam room effect.
- Sit in the steam for 10–20 minutes and practice breathwork, meditation, or lymphatic drainage.
- Bring in a bowl of boiling water and place a towel over your head (be careful!) to get targeted facial steam benefits.

## 3. SUN THERAPY (NATURE'S SAUNA)

- Spend 15–30 minutes outside in direct sunlight, allowing the body to heat naturally.
- Pair with light movement (like a walk or yoga) to amplify circulation and sweat.
- Sun exposure boosts vitamin D, enhances detoxification, and increases heat tolerance.

## 4. HOT BATH SOAK (DETOX + RELAXATION)

- Soak in a hot bath (around 100–105°F) for 20–30 minutes to induce sweating and muscle relaxation.
- Add Epsom salts, magnesium, or ginger powder to increase detox benefits and soothe sore muscles.
- Pair it with a cool rinse after to mimic contrast therapy.

## 5. WORKOUT IN A HOT ENVIRONMENT (INFRARED-FREE HEAT SHOCK THERAPY)

- Exercise in a warm room or wear extra layers to elevate core body temperature.
- Strength training, yoga, or cardio in a heated setting enhances endurance and heat adaptation.
- Afterward, cool down gradually to increase heat shock protein activation.

## 6. INTERNAL HEAT BOOST (SWEAT FROM THE INSIDE OUT)

- Drink hot herbal tea (ginger, cayenne, or turmeric-infused) to warm the body internally.
- Spicy foods (like capsaicin in chili peppers) increase body temperature and metabolism.
- Pair this with light movement or breathwork to intensify internal heat.

## 7. HEATED BLANKETS & LAYERING METHOD (OVERNIGHT HEAT THERAPY)

- Use an electric heating pad, heated blanket, or warm compress to increase local circulation.
- Sleeping in warmer conditions (but not too hot to disrupt sleep) can promote heat adaptation.
- Pair with hydration before bed to prevent dehydration from increased body temperature.

## 8. FAR-INFRARED HEATING PADS (MINI SAUNA BENEFITS WITHOUT THE PRICE TAG)

- Devices like BioMat or infrared heating pads provide targeted deep heat penetration.
- Great for muscle recovery, relaxation, and stimulating circulation without a full sauna setup.

## 9. HOT YOGA OR SWEAT-INDUCING WORKOUTS

- A hot yoga session mimics the effects of sauna exposure, increasing detoxification and flexibility.
- Even a regular workout with added clothing layers can help stimulate heat shock proteins and build heat resilience.

## 10. OUTDOOR HEAT EXPOSURE (HARNESS THE NATURAL WARMTH AROUND YOU)

- If you live in a warm climate, take advantage of the natural heat by sitting outside in the sun for 10–15 minutes.
- Opt for a shaded area if the sun is too intense, but allow your body to adjust to the heat gradually.
- Pair this with hydration, breathwork, or light stretching to enhance circulation and relaxation.
- This method helps acclimate your body to heat, improve tolerance, and stimulate heat shock proteins, without the need for expensive equipment.

## YOU DON'T NEED A SAUNA TO REAP THE BENEFITS!

Heat shock therapy doesn't require a high-end infrared setup. It's about consistency and using what's available. Whether you opt for a steamy shower, a hot bath, a sweaty workout, or simply basking in the sun, these small daily heat exposures can improve circulation, enhance detoxification, activate heat shock proteins, and boost overall wellbeing.

The key? Listen to your body, stack the habits that work for you, and make heat therapy part of your SUPERWELL routine!

---

> DON'T JUST CHECK THE BOXES.
> LIVE SUPERWELL AND
> *make it count.*

---

# COLD SHOCK THERAPY:

## MASTERING THE STRESS SWITCH

Cold exposure is more than just an extreme wellness trend—it's a scientifically backed method for building resilience, optimizing metabolism, and enhancing overall well-being. Cold shock therapy initiates a powerful physiological shift, moving the body from sympathetic (fight-or-flight) activation to parasympathetic (rest-and-digest) restoration. This ability to intentionally shift gears is a game-changer not just for the nervous system but for navigating stress in everyday life. By learning to get comfortable with the uncomfortable, you develop a skill set that translates beyond the plunge—into resilience, mental fortitude, and emotional stability.

When you first enter cold water, the body reacts with an immediate stress response. Blood vessels constrict, heart rate spikes, and norepinephrine surges. This is the sympathetic nervous system in action, priming you for survival. However, with intentional breathwork, you can override this automatic response, slowing the heart rate, deepening the breath, and shifting into a parasympathetic state. This conscious regulation of stress is a powerful skill that extends beyond the cold plunge and teaches you to manage daily pressures, anxiety, and emotional triggers with greater control.

### MENTAL RESILIENCE & STRESS ADAPTATION

Cold exposure forces the body to adapt to discomfort, making it a powerful tool for stress resilience. Studies show that repeated cold immersion lowers cortisol levels, improves stress tolerance, and enhances cognitive function. Just as strength training builds muscle, cold exposure strengthens mental fortitude, helping you develop a calmer, more controlled response to everyday stressors. Over time, the ability to breathe through discomfort in the plunge translates to better emotional regulation in real life.

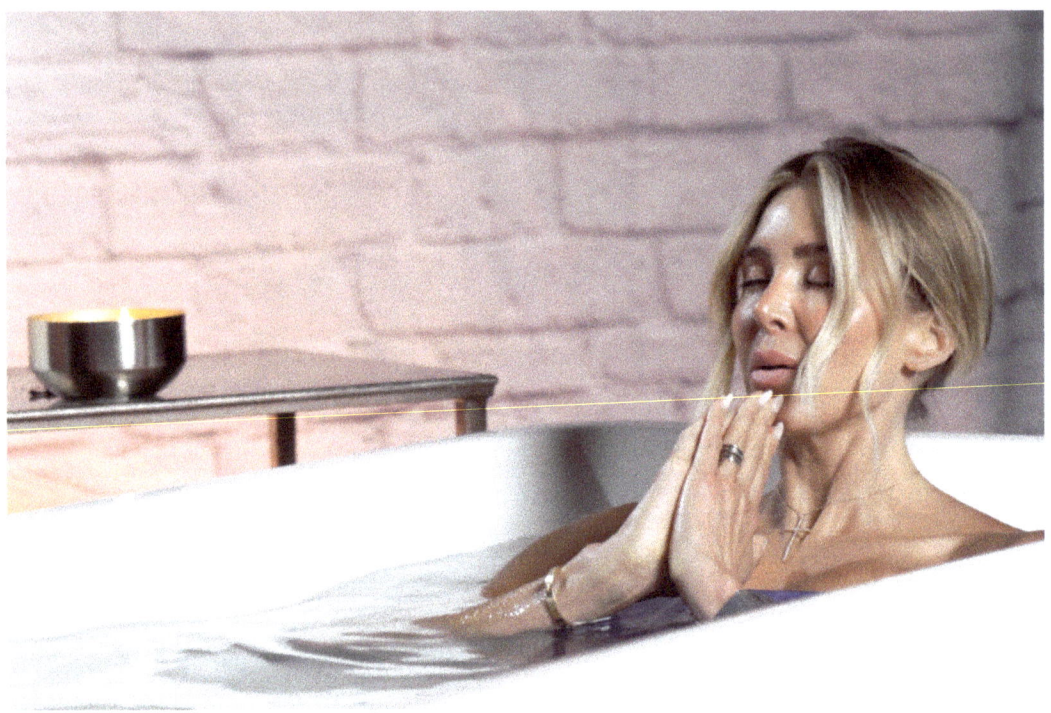

### RECOVERY & INFLAMMATION REDUCTION

Cold therapy is a game-changer for muscle recovery—reducing inflammation, flushing out metabolic waste, and accelerating healing post-exercise. The vasoconstriction (that is, blood vessel tightening) caused by cold exposure reduces swelling and lactic acid buildup, while the subsequent vasodilation (when warming up) floods tissues with oxygen-rich blood, aiding in faster muscle repair. Research has shown that regular cold plunges can cut post-workout soreness by up to 50%, making it a staple in elite athletic recovery protocols.

### METABOLIC BOOST & FAT ADAPTATION

Cold plunges activate brown adipose tissue (BAT), a metabolically active form of fat that burns energy to generate heat. This process, known as non-shivering thermogenesis, increases caloric expenditure, improves insulin sensitivity, and enhances metabolic flexibility. Regular exposure to cold has been shown to increase BAT activity, making the body more efficient at burning fat for energy. The result? Improved metabolic function, greater energy regulation, and enhanced endurance.

## NEUROCHEMICAL WAKE-UP CALL & ENERGY SURGE

The initial cold shock triggers a surge of norepinephrine, which is an alertness-boosting neurotransmitter that sharpens focus, heightens cognitive function, and elevates mood. Research shows that norepinephrine levels can increase by 200–300% with consistent cold exposure, leading to sustained mental clarity and heightened energy levels. This makes cold plunging an incredible natural stimulant without the crashes associated with caffeine or sugar.

## MOOD ELEVATION & MENTAL CLARITY

Cold water immersion is one of the fastest natural ways to boost dopamine levels, the neurotransmitter responsible for motivation, happiness, and cognitive performance. Studies show that a single cold plunge can increase dopamine by up to 250%—a longer-lasting effect than many antidepressants. Cold exposure also triggers the release of beta-endorphins, which reduce stress, enhance mood, and create a sense of post-plunge euphoria (yes, that happy, buzzing feeling after a cold dip is real!).

## MASTERING THE ART OF STRESS ADAPTATION

Cold shock therapy isn't just about braving the cold; it's about building resilience in every aspect of life. By learning to regulate stress responses, control breath, and stay present in discomfort, you train the body and mind to handle life's challenges with greater ease. Whether it's a cold plunge or a high-pressure situation, the ability to consciously shift your nervous system from a state of activation into one of calm and control is one of the most valuable skills you can cultivate.

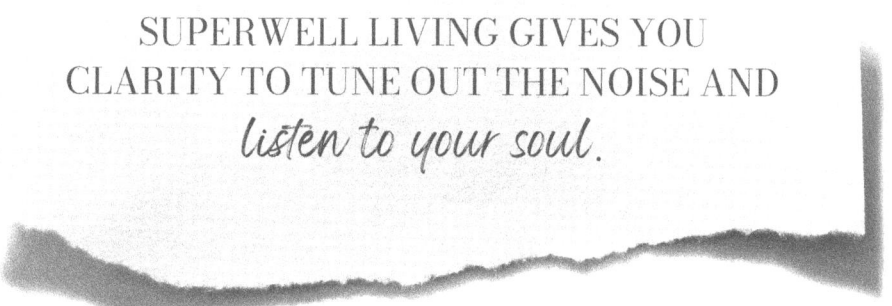

SUPERWELL LIVING GIVES YOU
CLARITY TO TUNE OUT THE NOISE AND
*listen to your soul.*

# 5 POWERFUL REASONS
## TO ACTIVATE YOUR BROWN FAT WITH COLD SHOCK

### BOOSTS METABOLISM & FAT BURNING

Brown fat activation generates heat through a process called thermogenesis, burning calories and increasing overall energy expenditure. This supports a healthy metabolism and can aid in weight management.

### ENHANCES INSULIN SENSITIVITY

Exposure to cold can improve insulin sensitivity, helping the body better regulate blood sugar levels. This reduces the risk of metabolic disorders like type 2 diabetes and promotes balanced energy levels.

### SUPPORTS HORMONAL BALANCE

Cold shock triggers the release of norepinephrine, a hormone and neurotransmitter that improves mood, focus, and alertness. It also helps reduce inflammation, enhancing overall hormonal health.

### IMPROVES MITOCHONDRIAL FUNCTION

Activating brown fat increases the activity and efficiency of mitochondria (the energy powerhouses of cells), supporting energy production and cellular health throughout the body.

### STRENGTHENS RESILIENCE AND STRESS RESPONSE

Cold exposure trains the body to handle stress more effectively by activating the sympathetic nervous system. This promotes better stress management, mental clarity, and emotional resilience in daily life.

## CREATIVE WAYS TO EXPERIENCE

# COLD SHOCK THERAPY
*(No Fancy Cold Tub Needed!)*

Cold shock therapy isn't just for those with high-end cold plunges. You can reap the benefits of cold exposure in creative, budget-friendly ways. Whether you want to ease into the cold or go all in, here are 10 ways to experience the power of cold shock therapy, no matter your setup.

### 1. COLD SHOWER METHOD (BEGINNER-FRIENDLY)

- Start with your usual warm shower, then gradually lower the temperature for the last 30–60 seconds.
- Over time, build up to 2–3 minutes of full cold exposure.
- Focus on breathing deeply to override the initial shock response.

### 2. ICE BOWL FACE DUNK (GREAT FOR LYMPHATIC DRAINAGE & MOOD BOOST)

- Fill a bowl with ice water and submerge your face for 15–30 seconds.
- Rest for 30 seconds, then repeat 2–3 times.
- Activates the mammalian dive reflex, lowering heart rate, reducing stress, and giving your skin a post-plunge glow.

## 3. DIY COLD TUB (FOR THOSE WHO WANT THE FULL-BODY PLUNGE WITHOUT THE PRICE TAG)

- Use a large storage bin or livestock water trough, filled with cold water and ice.
- If you have a bathtub, fill it with ice and water.
- Immerse yourself up to the neck.
- Try staying in for 2–5 minutes while controlling your breath.

## 4. CONTRAST THERAPY IN THE SHOWER (HOT-COLD CYCLING)

- Alternate between 30 seconds of cold water and 1 minute of warm water (repeat 3–4 cycles).
- This stimulates vascular expansion and contraction, improving circulation, immune function, and recovery.

## 5. COLD OUTDOOR EXPOSURE (NATURE'S FREE COLD THERAPY)

- Spend 10–15 minutes outside in cold temperatures wearing minimal layers.
- Great for activating brown fat, boosting metabolism, and building cold tolerance.
- Make it more fun by doing a walk, light workout, or breathwork session outside.

## 6. NATURAL WATER IMMERSION (FOR THOSE NEAR LAKES, RIVERS, OR THE OCEAN)

- Plunge into a cold lake, ocean, or river for a truly immersive cold shock experience.
- Nature adds an extra element of grounding and mental resilience.

## 7. ICE PACK METHOD (LOCALIZED COLD EXPOSURE)

- Apply an ice pack or frozen towel to the back of your neck, chest, or wrists.
- Helps activate the vagus nerve, reducing stress and improving mood.

## 8. CRYOTHERAPY ALTERNATIVE (COOLING YOUR BODY INTERNALLY)

- Drink ice-cold water or suck on ice chips to activate cold thermogenesis.
- Wearing a cooling vest or ice pack on your upper back also triggers cold adaptation.

## 9. COLD WORKOUT (TRAIN IN A CHILLED ENVIRONMENT)

- Lower your thermostat and exercise in a cold room or outside in cold weather.
- Training in the cold boosts calorie burn, improves endurance, and increases brown fat activation.

## 10. SLEEP COLD (FOR OVERNIGHT THERMOGENESIS)

- Lower your bedroom temperature to 60–67°F or sleep with fewer blankets.
- Sleeping in a cooler environment supports deeper sleep, metabolic health, and recovery.

## NO EXCUSES—THERE'S A COLD SHOCK OPTION FOR EVERYONE!

Cold therapy doesn't require an expensive plunge tub. It's about consistency, adaptation, and using the tools you have available. Whether you start with a cold shower, an ice bowl, or a winter walk, every small exposure builds your resilience, boosts your metabolism, and trains your body to handle stress more effectively. The key? Commit, breathe, and embrace the chill.

# GEAR SHIFTS TO SUPERWELL

## MASTERING YOUR NERVOUS SYSTEM WITH COLD SHOCK

One of the most powerful tools in my holistic toolkit and one that has profoundly impacted every aspect of my life is learning to control my central nervous system (CNS) through cold shock therapy. Whether in stressful situations, high-pressure business moments, or emotional challenges, the ability to intentionally shift my nervous system from overdrive to calm has been a game-changer.

The moment I submerge into 40-degree water, my sympathetic nervous system (fight-or-flight) kicks into full gear. Heart rate spikes, breath shortens, and my body sends signals of alarm, which is a primal reaction hardwired for survival. But here's where the magic happens: I have the power to override this automatic stress response.

Through controlled breathwork and intentional focus, I shift from stress overload into deep relaxation. Within 60 seconds, my body transitions into the parasympathetic nervous system (rest-and-digest), a state of calm, repair, and recovery. This shift isn't just about handling the cold. It's about training my nervous system to respond differently to all forms of stress in life.

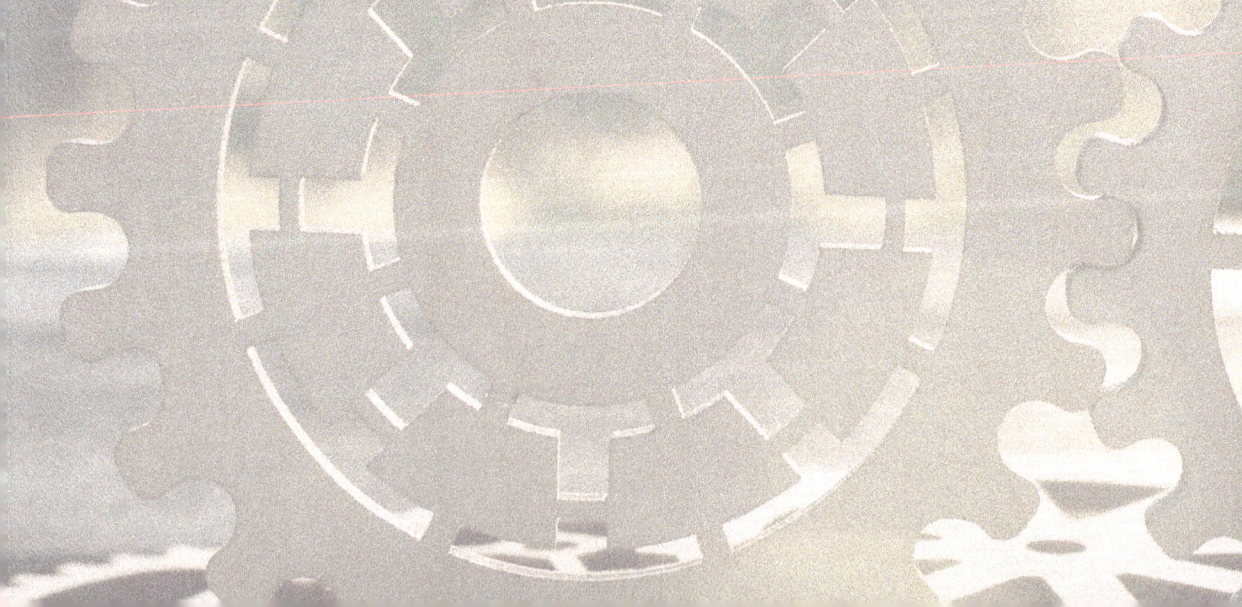

## BEYOND THE PLUNGE: TRAINING FOR LIFE'S CHALLENGES

Cold shock therapy isn't just about enduring icy waters—it's about commanding your body's physiological responses with precision. The ability to consciously shift from activation to restoration builds lasting resilience that extends far beyond the plunge.

Here's how I have applied CNS mastery to other areas of my life:

- **Business & Leadership** – Staying composed in high-stakes negotiations and high-pressure decisions
- **Parenting** – Responding to chaos with clarity rather than reacting impulsively
- **Public Speaking & Performance** – Regulating my breath and heart rate before stepping into the spotlight
- **Athletic & Physical Challenges** – Training my body to push beyond perceived limits without mental resistance
- **Emotional & Mental Resilience** – Shifting from anxiety and overwhelm to a state of calm and focus

Each cold plunge is a micro-dosage of controlled stress, training my system to adapt, recover, and respond with greater efficiency. It has rewired how I handle stress in everyday life, making me more present, focused, and unshakable under pressure.

## THE COLD AS A TEACHER

The practice of cold exposure teaches us that discomfort is temporary, fear is often an illusion, and we hold more control over our bodies than we realize. By repeatedly stepping into the cold, we train our nervous system to embrace stress, move through it, and release it, rather than being trapped in chronic overdrive.

This isn't just a wellness hack; it's a life mastery tool. The ability to regulate your nervous system at will is one of the greatest skills you can develop for both physical vitality and mental fortitude. Each plunge is more than just exposure—it's a step toward thriving in both health and life.

# HEAVY LIFTING
## STRENGTH UNLEASHED

Strength training is an indispensable pillar of SUPERWELL Living, especially for women seeking optimal health. Engaging in regular strength training, including lifting heavy weights, significantly enhances muscle mass, bone density, and metabolic rate. For women, this practice is crucial, as it counteracts the natural decline in muscle mass and bone density that occurs with age, reducing the risk of osteoporosis and sarcopenia. Furthermore, strength training boosts the production of growth hormones and accelerates fat loss, leading to a more toned physique and improved metabolic function. By incorporating heavy lifting into your routine, you not only build physical strength but also cultivate mental resilience and confidence. Embrace the power of strength training to achieve a balanced and empowered state of wellbeing.

### STRENGTH BUILDING

Strength training is vital for women because it boosts muscle mass and enhances bone density. Engaging in resistance exercises strengthens muscles and increases metabolism, while also stimulating bone-forming cells to improve bone density. This helps maintain bone health and prevent osteoporosis, supporting overall strength and vitality.

### METABOLISM BOOST

Strength training significantly boosts metabolic rate, helping with weight management by increasing the number of calories your body burns at rest. This elevated metabolism not only supports weight control but also enhances overall energy levels and promotes a leaner physique. As muscle mass increases, your body becomes more efficient at burning calories, making it easier to maintain or achieve a healthy weight.

## HEART HEALTH

Regular exercise is crucial for supporting cardiovascular health. Engaging in physical activity strengthens the heart, improves circulation, and helps maintain healthy blood pressure levels. It also enhances the efficiency of the cardiovascular system by increasing blood flow and reducing the risk of heart disease and stroke. Consistent exercise helps regulate cholesterol levels and promotes overall heart wellness, contributing to a healthier and more resilient cardiovascular system.

## MENTAL HEALTH

Exercise releases endorphins, which are natural mood enhancers that improve overall happiness and reduce stress. These "feel good" chemicals create a sense of wellbeing and euphoria, helping to alleviate anxiety and boost mental health. Regular physical activity not only supports emotional resilience but also contributes to a more positive and relaxed state of mind.

## LONGEVITY

Strength training contributes to a longer, healthier life by improving muscle mass, bone density, and overall functional fitness. It supports mobility, reduces the risk of chronic diseases, and enhances quality of life as you age.

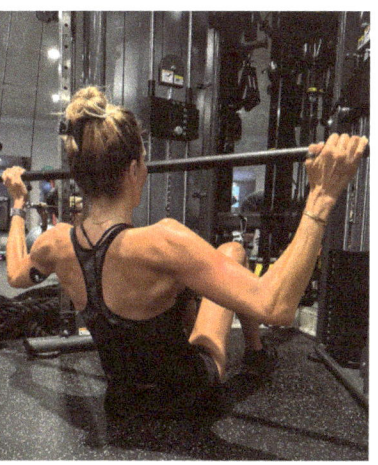
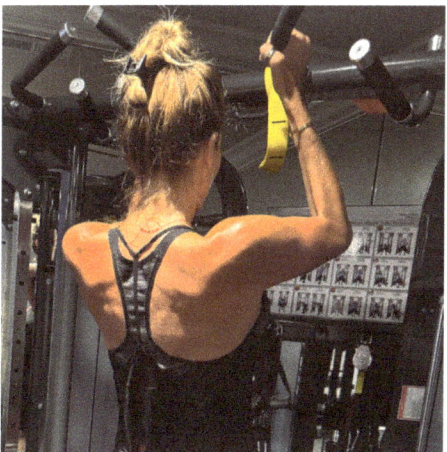
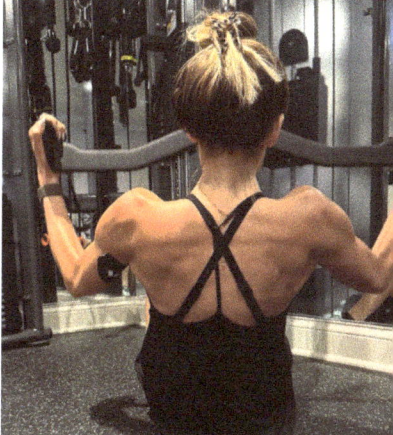

## The 20-Minute Momentum Hack:
# TRICK YOUR BRAIN, TRANSFORM YOUR DAY

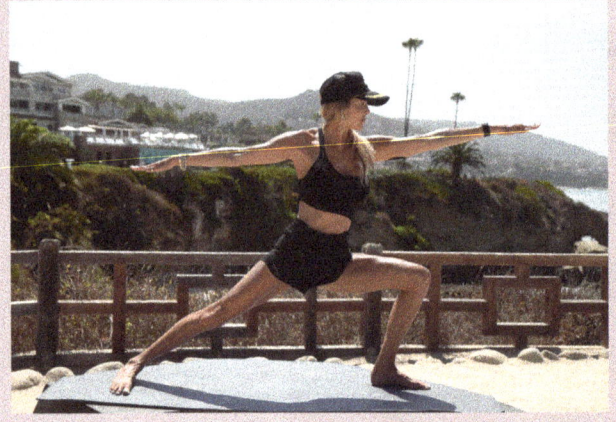
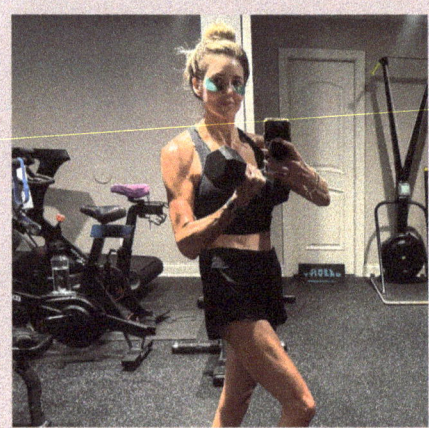

Some days, I wake up feeling totally unmotivated to move. My energy is low, my schedule is packed, and every excuse in the book sounds *completely valid*. But here's my secret weapon: I never let motivation be the deciding factor. Instead, I make a deal with myself: just 20 minutes. No pressure, no expectations. Maybe it's a quick walk outside, a Pilates flow, or some light strength work. Just enough to start.

And you know what happens? Nine times out of ten, that 20 minutes turns into an hour. Once I get moving, my energy shifts, my mindset clears, and suddenly, I remember why I do this. My stress melts, my focus sharpens, and my body thanks me with a surge of endorphins. I walk away feeling stronger, more centered, and completely reset, like I just flipped the switch on my day.

Because here's the truth: I have never, not once, regretted a workout. I have never finished a session and thought, *Wow, I really wish I hadn't moved my body today.* But on the days I skip? I feel the difference, with notably less energy, more stress, and a lingering sense of being "off."

Movement isn't just about exercise; it's about momentum. It's about honoring my body, clearing my mind, and reminding myself that even on my toughest days, I am in control of my energy. The hardest part is just starting. So, take the first step, commit to just 20 minutes, and let your body do the rest.

## Breaking Free from the Cardio Hamster Wheel:
# TRAIN SMARTER, NOT HARDER

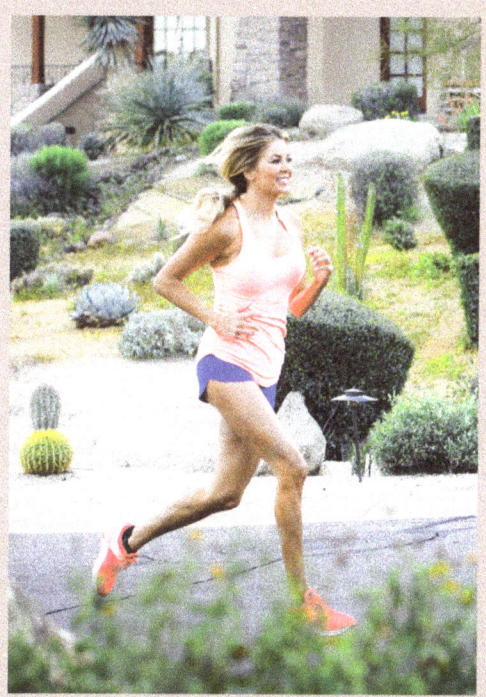

For years, I was a cardio bunny, running myself into the ground, literally. The elliptical, the treadmill, the spin classes—if it promised to burn calories, I was on it. And the result? I looked and felt my absolute worst. Puffy, inflamed, dark circles under my eyes, exhausted skin, chronically tired despite "doing everything right." My body was screaming *stop beating me up!* But I ignored the signs and kept pushing until I crashed headfirst into burnout hell.

That was my wake-up call. Cardio wasn't the answer—it was the problem. Overdoing it was spiking my cortisol, disrupting my hormones, and draining my energy instead of building it. So, I flipped the script and completely rewired my approach to movement. Now? I only practice true, intense cardio 2–3 times per week for just 5–8 minutes, because that's all you need to build a strong, resilient heart (yes, it's a muscle too!) and enhance cardiovascular health *without* sending your body into survival mode.

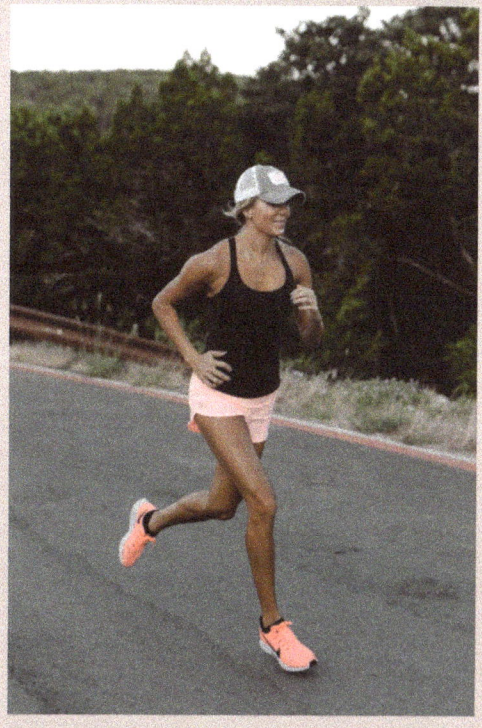

## How to Train Your Heart
# WITHOUT DESTROYING YOUR HORMONES

Instead of hours of soul-crushing cardio, I focus on short bursts of high-intensity, heart-strengthening work. Your heart needs to be trained like any other muscle, not overworked! Here's how I do it.

### 1. ECHO BIKE SPRINTS (AIR BIKE)
- 1-minute all-out sprint (push hard!)
- 1-minute slow recovery pace
- Repeat 5–8 times.
- Why? This targets both aerobic and anaerobic systems, improves VO2 max, and is low-impact but high-intensity.

### 2. TREADMILL SPRINT INTERVALS
- 1-minute all-out run (8–12 mph, depending on ability).
- 1-minute walk/recovery drift.
- Repeat 5–8 times.
- Why? Boosts mitochondrial efficiency, strengthens the heart, and burns fat without tanking your hormones.

### 3. INCLINE WALKING (POWER HILLS)
- Walk at 10–15% incline for 10–15 minutes at a brisk pace (3.5–4 mph).
- Why? Elevates heart rate without pounding the joints, improves leg strength and endurance, and supports lymphatic drainage.

### 4. SLED PUSHES OR FARMER'S CARRIES
- 30–60 seconds of sled pushing or heavy carries.
- Rest for 30–60 seconds.
- Repeat 4–6 rounds.
- Why? Full-body power and endurance training that challenges the heart and muscles simultaneously.

### 5. ROWING MACHINE POWER INTERVALS
- 30-second all-out row sprint.
- 30-second easy row recovery.
- Repeat 8–10 times.
- Why? Targets cardiovascular endurance, back strength, and explosive power without excessive impact.

## The Magic of Gentle Movement:
# TREAT YOUR BODY WITH KINDNESS

The harder I pushed myself with intense cardio, the worse I felt and looked. But when I slowed down by prioritizing Pilates, yoga, restorative movement, and walks in nature, my body responded beautifully. My energy came back, my inflammation vanished, my skin glowed again, and I finally felt strong and balanced.

The truth is, your body doesn't need constant punishment; it just needs support. Overdoing cardio isn't just exhausting; it's detrimental to female hormones. It increases cortisol, disrupts progesterone balance, and makes fat loss harder, not easier.

So here's my advice: Ditch the hamster wheel. Move with intention. Be kind to your body, and it will thank you. Because the goal isn't to break yourself down, it's to build yourself up.

# STRENGTH TRAINING FOR WOMEN & LONGEVITY

## KEY BENEFITS OF STRENGTH TRAINING

- **Improves Muscle Mass** – Maintains lean muscle as you age.
- **Stronger Bones** – Reduces the risk of osteoporosis and fractures.
- **Better Heart Health** – Enhances cardiovascular function.
- **Boosted Metabolism** – Increases resting metabolic rate, aiding weight management.

## LONGEVITY & DISEASE PREVENTION

- Reduces the risk of chronic diseases like diabetes, heart disease, and arthritis.
- Increases life expectancy: Studies show strength training may add years to your life.
- Helps manage and prevent obesity by increasing fat burning.

## MENTAL HEALTH & COGNITIVE FUNCTION

- Improves mood and reduces symptoms of depression.
- Enhances brain function and reduces cognitive decline.

## PRACTICAL TIPS FOR WOMEN

- Start light and gradually increase weights.
- Aim for 2–3 strength training sessions per week.
- Include compound exercises (e.g., squats, deadlifts, lunges).

# STRENGTH IS YOUR SUPERPOWER

Strength training isn't just about muscle—it's a prescription for longevity. For women, it's one of the most effective ways to extend healthspan, boost metabolism, balance hormones, sharpen cognitive function, and preserve independence as we age. It builds resilience from the inside out—supporting your bones, brain, and nervous system while helping you feel empowered in your own skin.

**Pro Tip:** For optimal results, pair strength training with 30 grams of protein per meal, daily creatine, and post-workout recovery like cold immersion or red light therapy. These strategies supercharge muscle repair, regulate hormones, and unlock cellular rejuvenation.

Lift smart. Recover well. Live SUPERWELL.

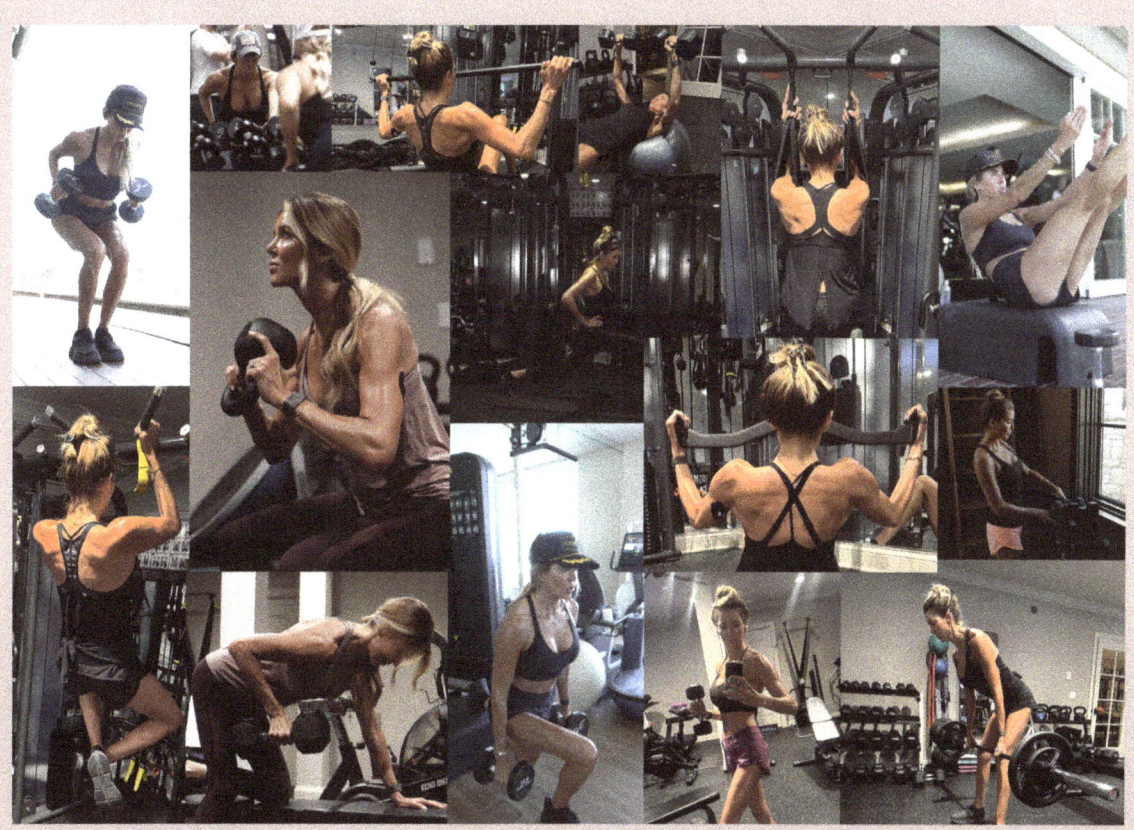

# THE BEGINNER'S GUIDE TO STRENGTH TRAINING FOR WOMEN'S LONGEVITY

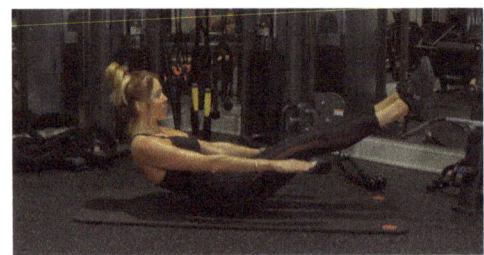

**THE HUNDRED**

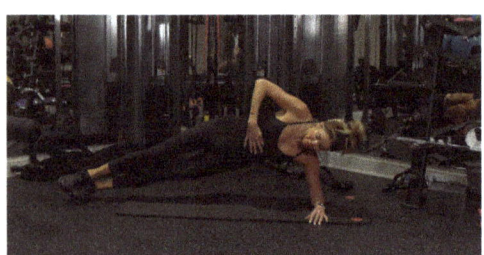

**SIDE PLANK WITH KNEE TAP**

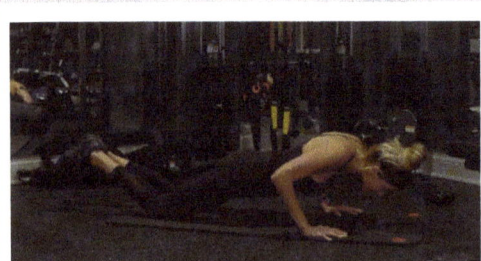

**REGULAR OR MODIFIED PUSH-UPS**

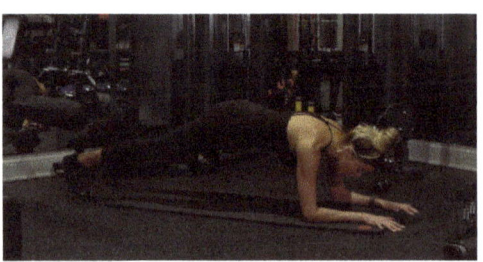

**FOREARM PLANK**

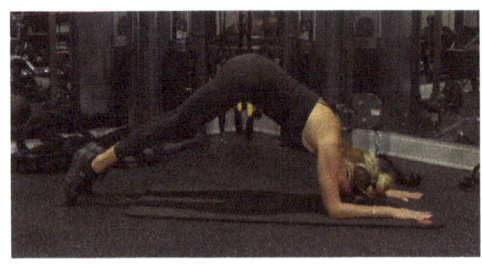

**PLANK TO DOLPHIN**

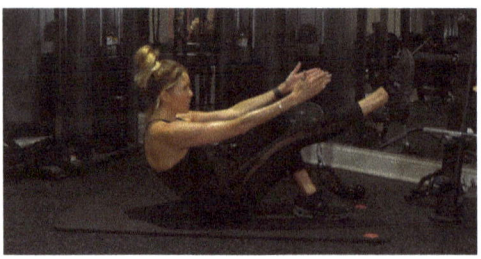

**SINGLE-LEG CIRCLES**

# The Beginner's Guide to Strength Training | 113

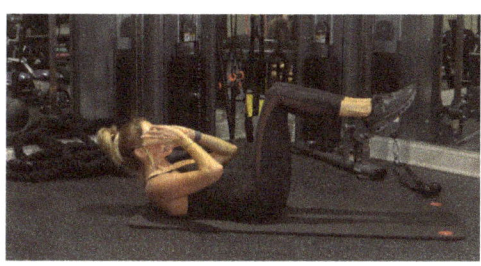

**DOUBLE-LEG STRETCH**

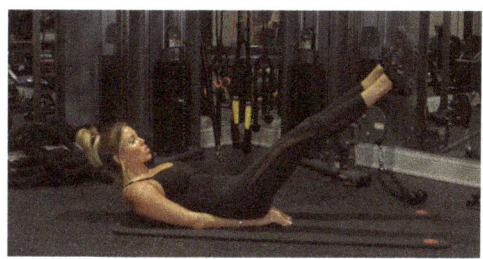

**DOUBLE-LEG CIRCLES**

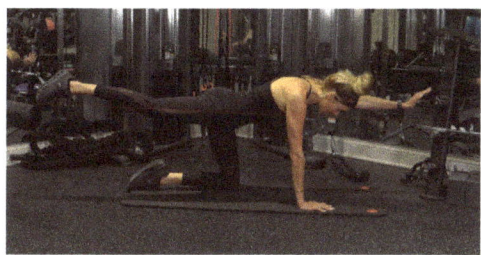

**BIRD-DOG PLANK**

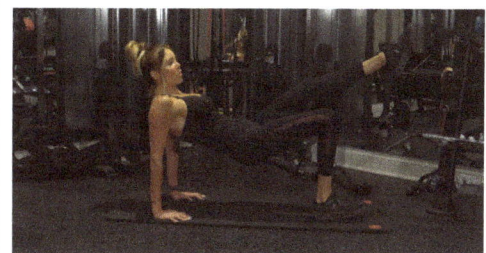

**REVERSE PLANK WITH KNEE TUCKS**

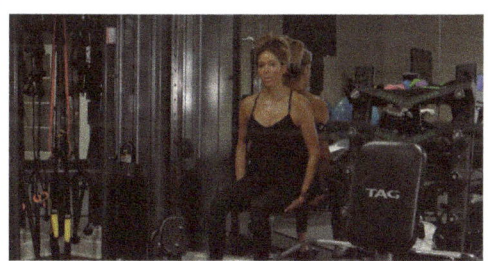

**WALL SIT WITH OR WITHOUT DUMBBELLS**

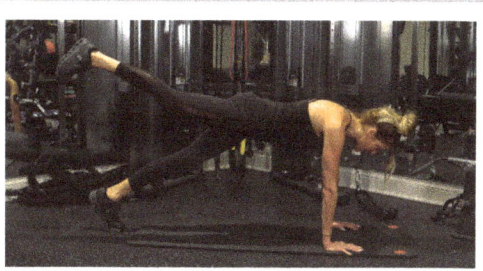

**PLANK LEG LIFT**

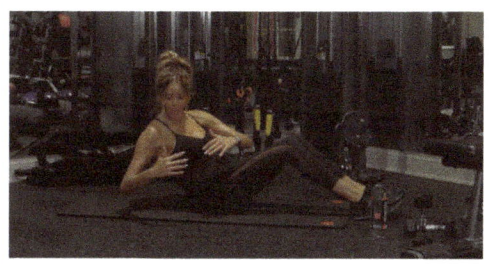

**RUSSIAN TWISTS**

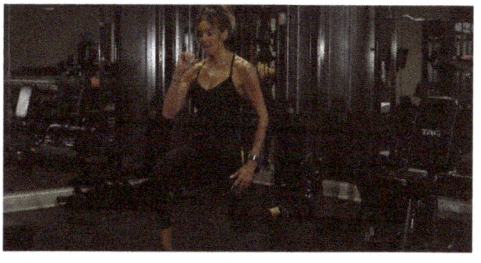

**FORWARD LUNGES**

# ESSENTIAL STRETCHES
## FOR RELAXATION & FLEXIBILITY

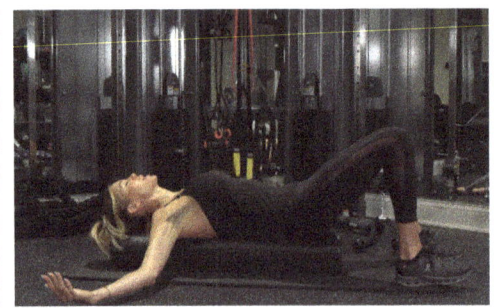

**SPINE ROLLER**

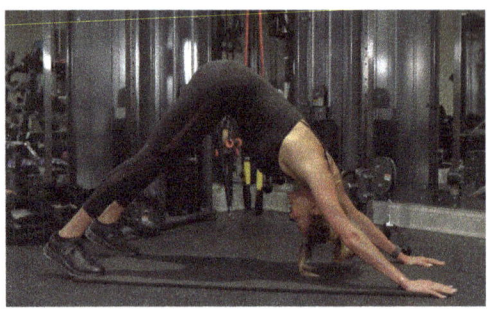

**DOWNWARD DOG**

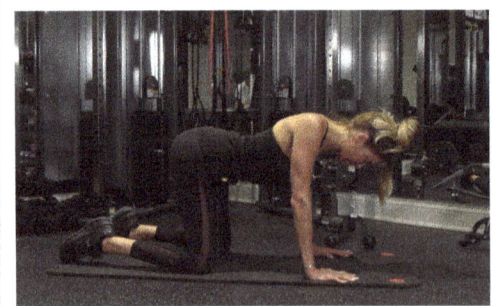

**CAT-COW STRETCH**

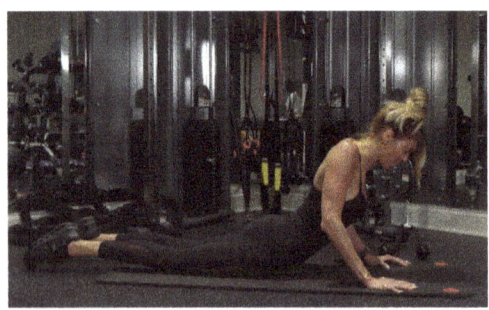

**COBRA STRETCH**

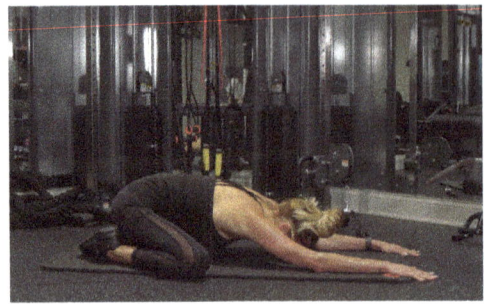

**CHILD'S POSE**

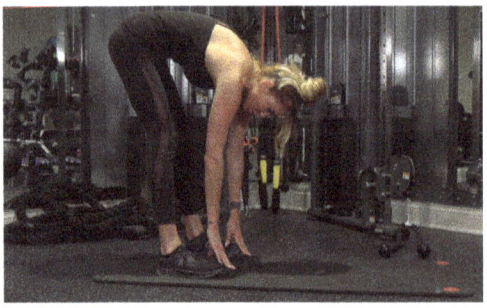

**STANDING FORWARD FOLD**

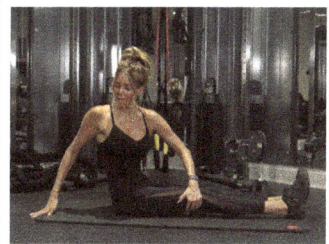
SEATED SPINAL TWIST

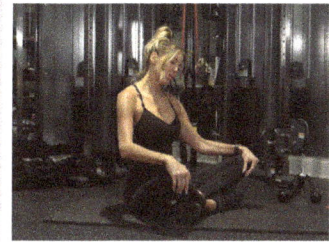
NECK ROLLS

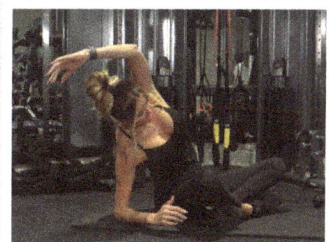
SIDE BODY STRETCH

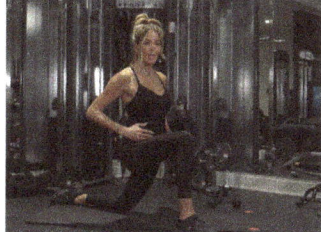
HIP FLEXOR STRETCH

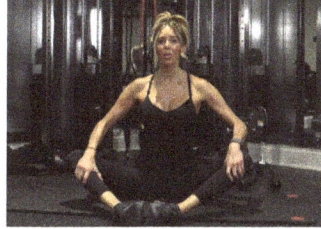
BUTTERFLY STRETCH

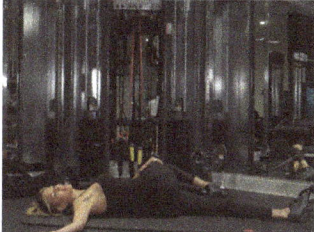
LUMBAR ROTATION STRETCH

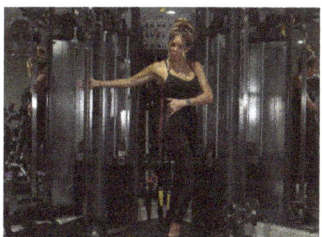
CHEST OPENER STRETCH

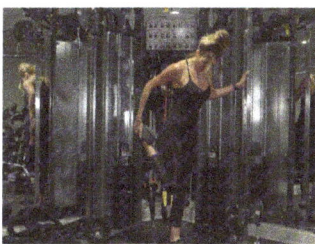
BASIC QUAD STRETCH

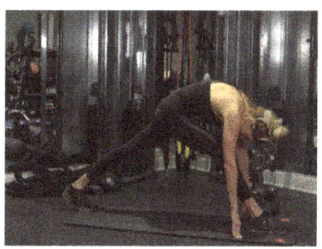
BASIC RUNNER'S LUNGE

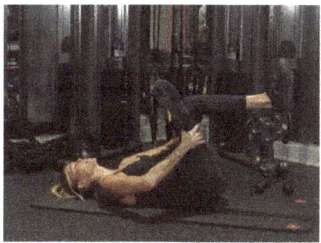
FIGURE FOUR STRETCH

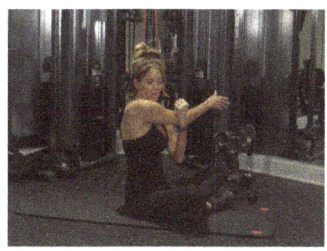
ARM ACROSS CHEST STRETCH

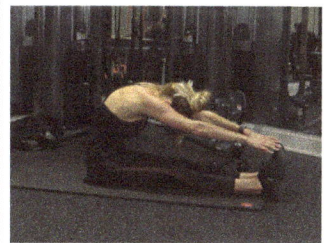
SEATED TOE TOUCH

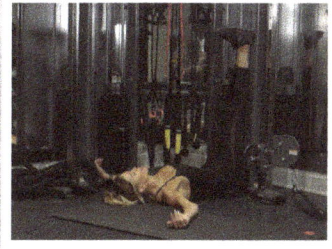
LEGS UP THE WALL

YOUR JOURNEY TO SUPERWELL STARTS WITH ONE SMALL, *intentional step today.*

# BASIC MAT
# PILATES EXERCISES

*In Pilates, form is everything.* Less is more; think quality over quantity. Breathe with intention, move with control, and remember: Your *powerhouse* is not just your abs, it's your entire core system, from shoulders to hips.

Let these 10 movements be your foundation for building a resilient, flexible, and strong body because when your core is strong, everything else follows.

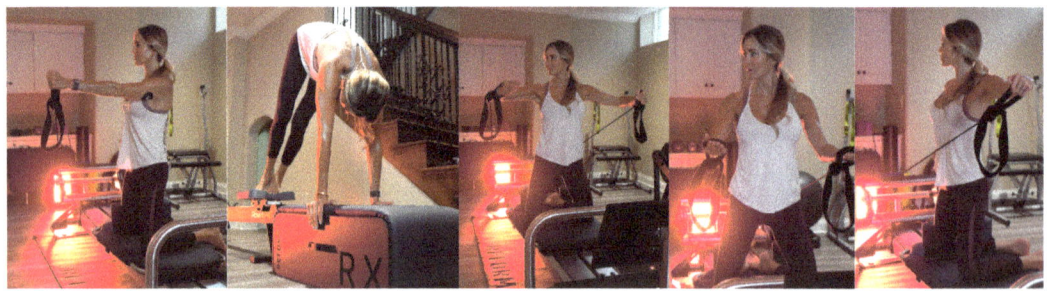

## 1. THE HUNDRED

**HOW TO:**
Lie on your back, legs lifted to tabletop or extended straight at a 45° angle. Lift your head, neck, and shoulders off the mat, arms reaching long beside you. Pump the arms up and down with small, controlled movements as you inhale for 5 counts and exhale for 5 counts. Repeat for 10 full breaths (100 arm pumps).

**BENEFITS:**
- Activates deep core muscles (transverse abdominis).
- Increases circulation and breath control.
- Warms up the body and mind for the rest of your practice.

## 2. SINGLE-LEG STRETCH

### HOW TO:
Lie on your back, knees to chest. Lift head and shoulders, hold right shin, extend left leg at a 45° angle. Switch legs, pulling the opposite knee in.

### BENEFITS:
- Improves spinal stability.
- Strengthens the abdominals and hip flexors.
- Teaches controlled movement while engaging the core.

## 3. DOUBLE-LEG STRETCH

### HOW TO:
Start in the same position as the single-leg stretch. Inhale as you reach both arms overhead and extend both legs out at a 45° angle. Exhale as you circle the arms back to the knees and return to the start.

### BENEFITS:
- Builds deep core strength and coordination.
- Protects the back by training pelvic stability.
- Increases endurance and control.

## 4. ROLL-UP

### HOW TO:
Lie flat with arms overhead. Inhale, lift arms, head, and spine off the mat one vertebra at a time. Exhale as you reach toward your toes. Inhale to begin rolling back down slowly.

### BENEFITS:
- Increases spinal mobility and articulation.
- Strengthens the abdominals more effectively than traditional sit-ups.
- Teaches control through full range of motion.

## 5. SINGLE-LEG CIRCLES

HOW TO:

Lie on your back, one leg extended on the mat, the other leg lifted straight up. Circle the raised leg across the body, down, and around without shifting your pelvis. Perform 5 in each direction.

BENEFITS:
- Strengthens the core through stabilization.
- Mobilizes the hip joint.
- Teaches pelvic control and coordination.

## 6. PLANK TO LEG LIFT

HOW TO:

Start in a forearm or full plank position. Engage your core and glutes as you lift one leg off the ground, keeping hips stable. Alternate legs slowly.

BENEFITS:
- Strengthens shoulders, abdominals, and glutes.
- Promotes spinal alignment.
- Builds full-body endurance and stability.

## 7. SIDE-LYING LEG LIFTS

HOW TO:

Lie on one side, legs extended and stacked. Rest your head on your lower arm. Lift and lower the top leg with control. Keep the core tight to avoid rocking.

BENEFITS:
- Strengthens obliques, hips, and outer thighs.
- Supports pelvic alignment and spinal protection.
- Enhances balance and muscular symmetry.

## 8. THE SAW

**HOW TO:**

Sit tall with legs extended wider than hip-width, arms outstretched. Inhale to twist toward one leg, exhale to reach pinky finger toward pinky toe with a sawlike motion. Return to center and switch.

**BENEFITS:**
- Increases spinal rotation and hamstring flexibility.
- Engages obliques and deep core.
- Encourages postural awareness.

## 9. SWIMMING

**HOW TO:**

Lie face down, arms extended overhead. Lift arms, chest, and legs slightly off the mat. Flutter arms and legs in a swimming motion while keeping the core engaged.

**BENEFITS:**
- Strengthens posterior chain (back, glutes, shoulders).
- Improves coordination and spinal extension.
- Enhances back-body awareness.

## 10. PELVIC CURL (BRIDGE)

**HOW TO:**

Lie on your back, knees bent, feet hip-width apart. Inhale, then exhale to lift the pelvis one vertebra at a time until the hips are lifted. Inhale at the top, then exhale as you roll down slowly.

**BENEFITS:**
- Strengthens glutes and hamstrings.
- Improves spinal articulation and pelvic control.
- Supports low back stability and flexibility.

# 10 Benefits of
# PILATES MOVEMENT

### 1. CORE STRENGTH & STABILITY

Pilates is renowned for building deep core strength, targeting muscles that support the spine and pelvis. A strong core improves posture, balance, and overall movement efficiency, reducing the risk of back pain and injury.

### 2. ENHANCED FLEXIBILITY & MOBILITY

Unlike static stretching, Pilates incorporates dynamic flexibility, allowing muscles to lengthen while maintaining strength and control. This approach improves range of motion in the spine, hips, and hamstrings, leading to better functional movement and reduced stiffness.

### 3. POSTURE PERFECTION & SPINAL HEALTH

By focusing on alignment and controlled movements, Pilates strengthens postural muscles, preventing the slouched shoulders and forward-head posture caused by modern lifestyles. A properly aligned spine reduces strain on joints and enhances breathing efficiency.

### 4. LEAN MUSCLE TONE WITHOUT BULK

Pilates lengthens and strengthens muscles simultaneously, creating a lean, sculpted physique without excessive bulk. By engaging stabilizing muscles, it enhances definition while maintaining flexibility and fluid movement.

### 5. STRESS RELIEF & NERVOUS SYSTEM REGULATION

Through focused breathing and mindful movement, Pilates activates the parasympathetic nervous system (rest-and-digest), reducing cortisol levels and promoting a state of calm. This mind-body connection enhances mental clarity and emotional resilience.

## 6. INJURY PREVENTION & JOINT SUPPORT

Pilates is a low-impact, joint-friendly practice that builds balanced muscle strength, reducing strain on knees, hips, and lower back. By enhancing mobility and stabilization, it minimizes the risk of overuse injuries common in high-impact workouts.

## 7. FUNCTIONAL STRENGTH & EVERYDAY PERFORMANCE

Pilates trains the body in multi-directional, real-life movements, improving strength for daily activities like lifting, bending, and reaching. By activating smaller stabilizing muscles, it enhances overall coordination and efficiency in movement.

## 8. IMPROVED ATHLETIC PERFORMANCE

Many elite athletes incorporate Pilates to enhance flexibility, strength, and injury prevention. The focus on core engagement, spinal mobility, and muscle endurance improves explosive power, balance, and movement efficiency in sports performance.

## 9. BETTER CIRCULATION & DETOXIFICATION

Controlled, fluid movements stimulate blood flow and lymphatic drainage, helping to flush toxins and reduce inflammation. The deep breathing techniques used in Pilates oxygenate the blood, enhancing cellular regeneration and overall vitality.

## 10. HORMONAL BALANCE & SUSTAINABLE FITNESS

Unlike high-intensity workouts that spike cortisol, Pilates is a hormone-friendly way to stay strong without overtaxing the body. By combining strength, flexibility, and controlled breathing, it supports hormonal equilibrium, making it an ideal movement practice for women's health and longevity.

---

THE SUPERWELL METHOD INVITES YOU TO
*be consistent, not perfect.*

# GLUCOSE GARBAGE DUMP

## GLUCOSE & INSULIN REGULATION:

**What Happens Without Exercise?** – When we don't move enough, glucose remains in the bloodstream, leading to higher blood sugar levels.

**How Exercise Helps** – Physical activity improves insulin sensitivity, allowing glucose to enter muscle cells more effectively for energy, reducing excess glucose in the bloodstream.

## THE "GLUCOSE GARBAGE DUMP" CONCEPT

**Muscle Activity** – During exercise, muscles act as a "glucose dump" by taking in glucose from the blood. This helps prevent glucose from accumulating and causing spikes in blood sugar.

**HIIT and Strength Training** – High-intensity interval training (HIIT) and strength training workouts are particularly effective because they engage large muscle groups and require more glucose for energy, speeding up the clearance process.

## KEY BENEFITS:

**Improved Insulin Sensitivity** – Regular movement reduces the body's resistance to insulin, improving how glucose is processed.

**Fat Burning** – When glucose levels drop, the body taps into fat stores for energy, supporting fat loss.

**Enhanced Metabolism** – Exercise helps balance glucose and supports long-term metabolic health.

Incorporating regular physical activity into your routine is an effective way to manage blood sugar levels and promote overall metabolic health. The SUPERWELL Workout concept of using exercise as a "glucose garbage dump" demonstrates how movement can clear excess glucose from the bloodstream, improving insulin sensitivity, burning fat, and enhancing your body's metabolic efficiency.

# LAUREN'S SUPERWELL PEP TALK

## *Encouragement & Tips to Get You Moving!*

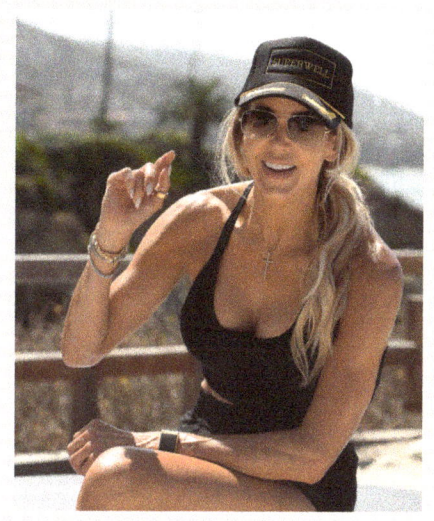

Movement isn't about perfection or pressure; it's about feeling good, building energy, and living fully. Here are some words straight from my heart to yours to help you make movement a joyful part of your life.

### 1. ACTION CHANGES EVERYTHING

Sometimes the hardest part is starting. Take that first step, whether it's a short walk, a stretch, taking a class, or doing a dance in your living room. Every little bit counts.

### 2. MAKE IT FUN

Movement doesn't have to feel like "exercise." Dance, play with your kids, hike, or simply move to your favorite playlist. When you enjoy it, you will keep coming back for more.

### 3. CELEBRATE YOUR BODY

Your body is incredible and it carries you through life every day. Move because you love it, not because you are trying to punish it. Every step forward is progress.

### 4. IT'S NOT ABOUT TIME; IT'S ABOUT CONSISTENCY

Even 20 minutes of movement can boost your energy and mood. It's not about doing it all; it's about showing up for yourself, day after day.

### 5. MOVEMENT IS FREEDOM

When you move, you clear your mind, fuel your soul, and unlock a sense of freedom. Let movement remind you of your strength and power.

You deserve to feel amazing. Move for yourself. Live SUPERWELL.

# SUPERWELL TAKEAWAYS

### STRONG WOMEN AGE DIFFERENTLY

- Bones shrink, metabolism slows, and hormones shift, but strength training rewrites the script.
- It builds bone density, preserves lean muscle, balances hormones, and boosts metabolic health.
- Muscle doesn't make you bulky. It makes you bulletproof.

### MUSCLE IS YOUR METABOLIC ENGINE

- More muscle = more calories burned at rest.
- Stop chasing calorie deficits and start building your burn.
- Strength training turns your body into a 24/7 fat-burning machine.

### MUSCLE IS MEDICINE

- Strength training improves insulin sensitivity, lowers inflammation, and sharpens brain function.
- It's not just about aesthetics—it's your prescription for disease prevention.
- Muscle is anti-aging, anti-diabetes, anti-anxiety . . . and pro-*power*.

### STRONG IS A MINDSET

- Reps and sets build more than muscle—they build resilience.
- Each deadlift, lunge, and push-up trains your nervous system to handle stress.
- Train your body, strengthen your mind. The gym is your daily classroom for life mastery.

### BUILD STRENGTH FOR THE BODY YOU WANT TO LIVE IN

- You don't get the body you want by wishing—you earn it through consistency.
- Strength is built in the moments you don't quit.
- Your body is your home. Make it strong, capable, and fiercely independent.

### LIFT HEAVY. LIVE LONGER.

- Muscle mass is the #1 predictor of healthspan.
- Want to play on the floor with your grandkids at 80? Then pick up those weights now.

### THE REAL GLOW-UP? STRENGTH.

- Skin care gives you glow. Strength gives you power.
- Confidence hits different when it's backed by muscle.
- Lift heavy. Stand taller. Radiate strength from the inside out.

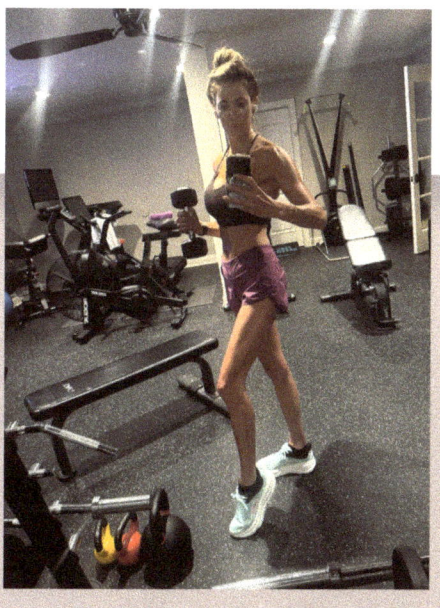
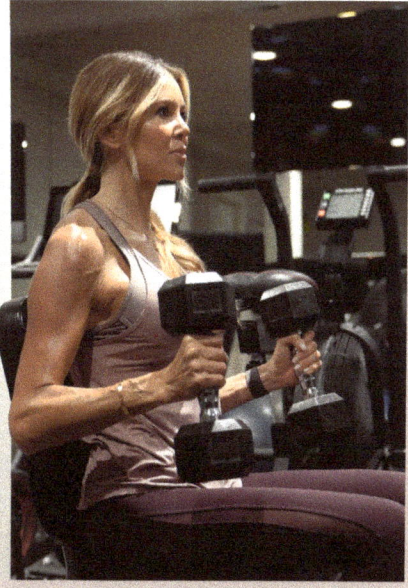

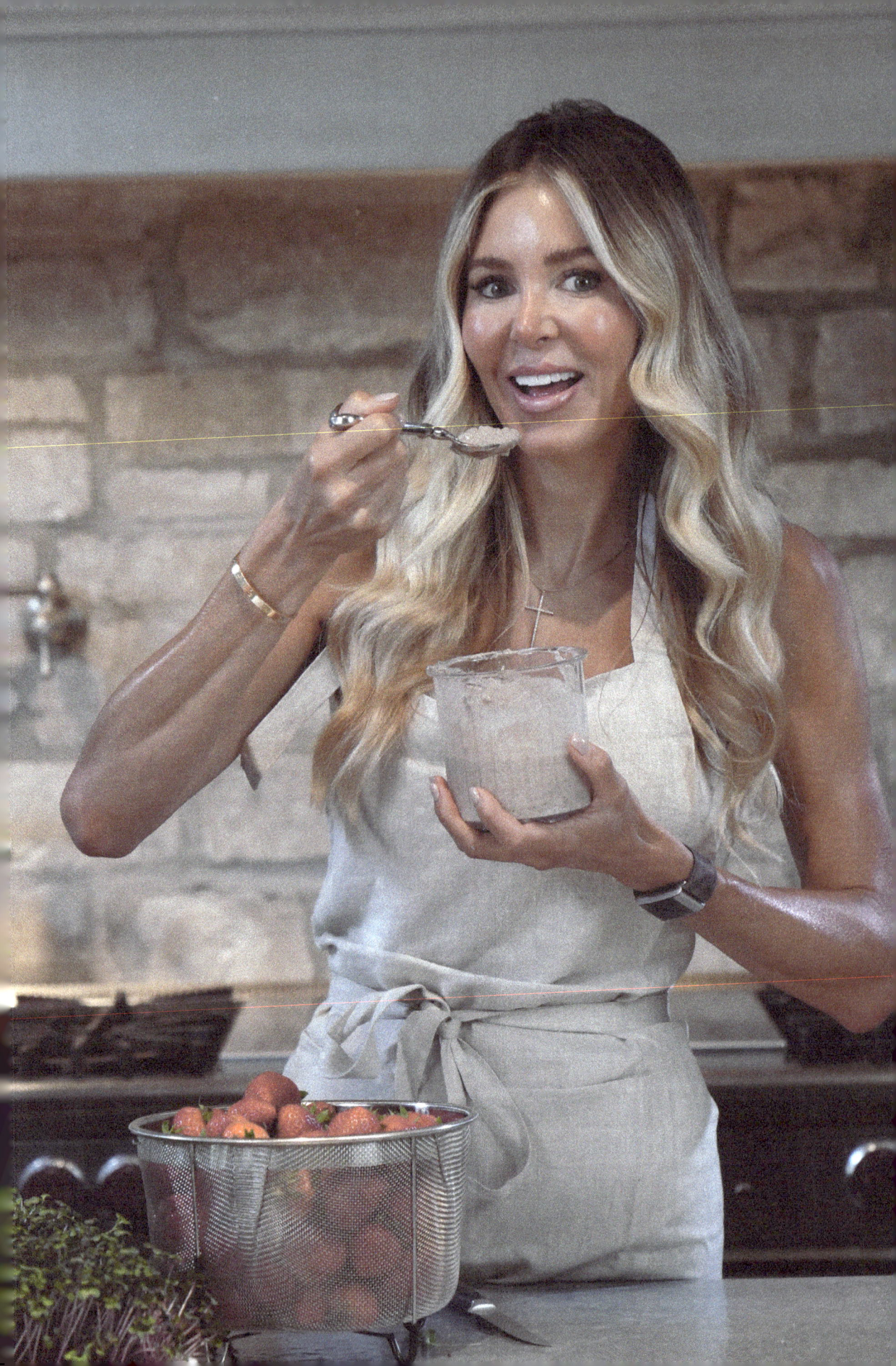

## THE SUPERWELL

# 12-INGREDIENT POWER PROTEIN MILKSHAKE

*Functional Fuel for Recovery, Digestion, & Daily Optimization*

Post-workout nutrition is not just about protein; it's about creating the ideal internal environment for muscle protein synthesis, metabolic regulation, and cellular repair. My signature SUPERWELL 12-Ingredient Power Protein Milkshake was born from years of trials and errors (always being the guinea pig). It's a powerhouse blend specifically formulated to support post-exercise recovery, regulate hormones, balance blood sugar, and feed the body on a cellular level.

Every ingredient serves a purpose. The high-quality complete protein (typically 20–30 g) activates mTOR pathways, essential for muscle repair and hypertrophy. Ingredients rich in micronutrients, antioxidants, omega-3s, prebiotics, and adaptogens support everything from mitochondrial health and immune resilience to gut-brain axis function and cognitive performance. This isn't just a "shake"—it's a biohacking upgrade in a cup.

# WHY IT WORKS: A DEEPER LOOK AT THE BENEFITS

## MUSCLE RECOVERY + GROWTH

Post-exercise, your muscles are in a catabolic state. The inclusion of complete protein sources, particularly those rich in leucine (an anabolic trigger), kickstarts muscle protein synthesis. I always aim for 1 gram of protein per pound of body weight, or more, depending on training load, because protein is also the foundation of enzymatic function, hormonal balance, and tissue repair. This shake ensures that my body rebuilds stronger, not just recovers.

## COGNITIVE + MENTAL PERFORMANCE

Many of the ingredients, such as healthy fats, greens, omega-3s, and adaptogenic herbs, help stabilize blood glucose and fuel the brain with clean-burning energy. Balanced blood sugar = stable mood, sharper focus, and better decision-making throughout the day.

## METABOLIC RESILIENCE

The strategic combination of protein + fiber + fat ensures a slow, sustained release of glucose, avoiding blood sugar spikes and crashes. This supports insulin sensitivity, cortisol regulation, and a feeling of steady, calm energy. It also supports satiety and fat metabolism by reducing cravings and overeating later in the day.

## GUT + IMMUNE SYSTEM SUPPORT

Over 70% of the immune system resides in the gut, and this shake includes prebiotic fiber, anti-inflammatory compounds, and digestive support (like ginger, greens, or probiotic powders). These ingredients help reinforce the intestinal lining, reduce bloat, and support a diverse and resilient gut microbiome, which in turn fuels your immune and mental health.

## HORMONAL + CELLULAR HEALTH

Including fiber, healthy fats, and detox-supportive greens helps clear excess estrogen and environmental toxins through improved liver and digestive function. Fiber also binds to cholesterol and supports cardiovascular health while feeding your beneficial gut flora, a win-win.

This shake isn't just delicious—it's a daily act of self-care, performance enhancement, and longevity insurance. It's the fuel that supports my strength training, keeps my skin glowing, and powers me through intense days without the crash. It's spoon-worthy, nutrient-dense, and wildly effective because you deserve to feel strong, nourished, and SUPERWELL from the inside out.

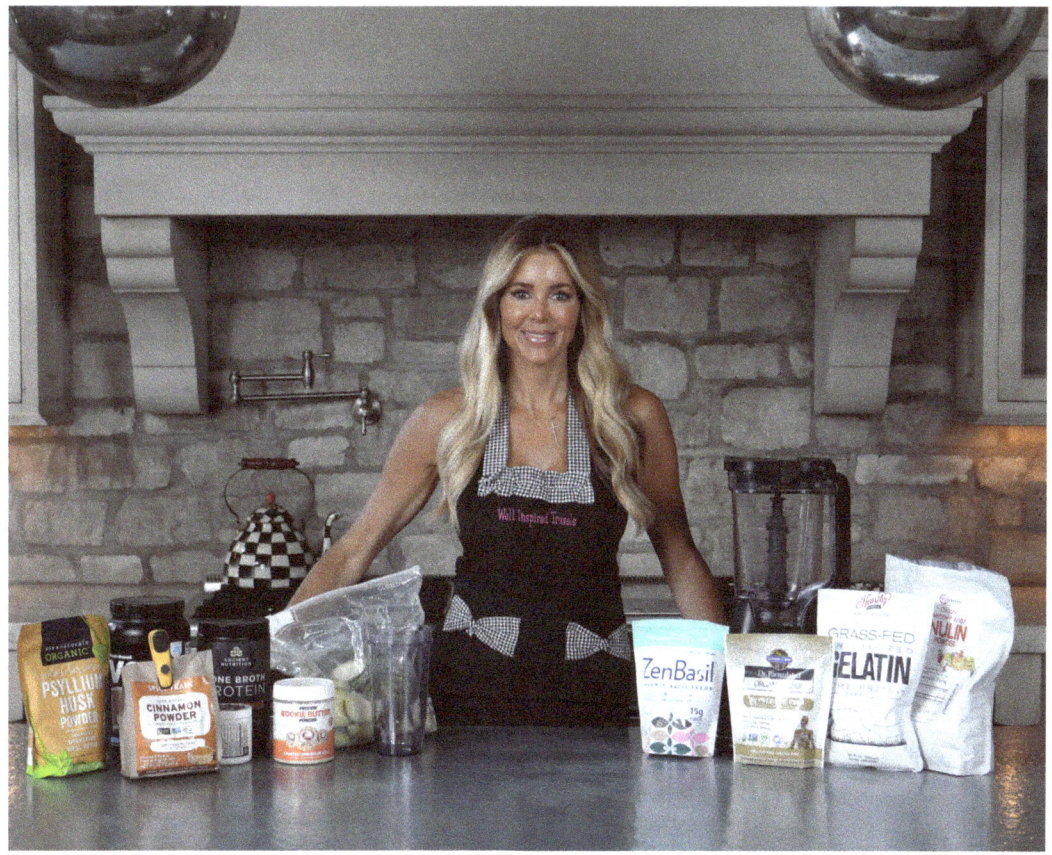

# LAUREN'S 12-INGREDIENT POWER
# *Protein Milkshake*

**YIELD: 2 SERVINGS**

Before you dive into the ingredients, it's important to understand: This is more than just a post-workout shake; this is a strategic metabolic reset and cellular nourishment tool. Designed to support muscle recovery, hormonal balance, gut integrity, and blood sugar stability, every ingredient in this SUPERWELL 12-Ingredient Power Protein Milkshake has a functional role. From collagen peptides to promote connective tissue repair to omega-rich seeds and adaptogenic mushroom blends that reduce inflammation and optimize brain function, this shake is your daily foundation for performance, clarity, and resilience.

Whether consumed after strength training or as a balanced start to your day, it supports both short-term recovery and long-term vitality.

- 2 tablespoons Zen Basil seeds
- 1/2 cup filtered water or milk of choice (for soaking)
- 10–12 ounces unsweetened vanilla almond milk, divided
- 1/2 cup (1 scoop) vanilla Vega Premium Sport Protein or your favorite choice of protein powder (I recommend a clean whey protein, if you don't have allergies), divided
- 1/2 cup (1 scoop) Ancient Nutrition salted caramel bone broth protein, divided
- 1–2 tablespoons Garden of Life organic fiber, divided (see note)
- 1 tablespoon Host Defense Stamets 7 mushroom powder, divided
- 1 tablespoon Hearthy Foods beef gelatin, divided
- 1 tablespoon Viva Naturals organic psyllium husk, divided
- 1 tablespoon SPICE TRAIN cinnamon powder, divided
- 1 tablespoon whey protein frosted cinnamon roll cookie butter powder, divided
- 1 tablespoon Pure Encapsulations L-Glutamine, divided
- 1–2 cups frozen sliced organic zucchini

1. In a covered glass jar, soak the Zen Basil seeds overnight in the filtered water (or milk of choice for extra creaminess). This enhances the seeds' bioavailability and transforms them into a gut-loving, fiber-rich gel for smoother digestion and better texture.

2. Line up all your ingredients for quick, seamless blending. Having everything pre-measured and within reach ensures nutrient retention and saves precious time.

3. Follow these SUPERWELL blending directions for maximum creaminess and efficiency. Strategic layering is key to achieving that perfectly creamy, frosty consistency, especially when using a high-powered blender like a Vitamix or Ninja BL610 Professional Plus. Here's how to layer it:

   - Base layer (wet): Start with half of your almond milk and soaked Zen Basil seeds.
   - Mid layer (dry): Add half of your dry ingredients (protein powders, fiber, mushroom powder, gelatin, psyllium husk, cinnamon, whey protein, and L-glutamine).
   - Hydration layer (wet): Pour in the remaining half of the almond milk.
   - Final layer (frozen): Top with your frozen sliced organic zucchini. This acts as the natural thickener and chill factor.

4. Begin on low speed and gradually increase to high. Blend for 30–60 seconds or until smooth and spoon-worthy.

### PRO TIP
- If blending stalls or thickens too much, pause and stir gently with a spoon or spatula. Add a splash of water or almond milk to adjust consistency, then reblend.

5. Pour and thrive! Enjoy immediately for post-workout recovery or as a high-performance meal foundation. It's creamy, satiating, and rich in nutrients that nourish your gut, support muscle repair, and fuel your SUPERWELL lifestyle.

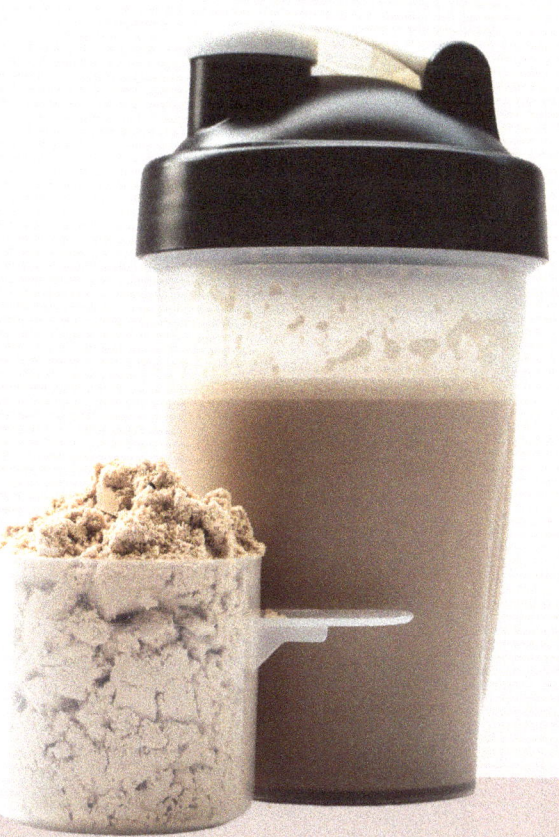

# THE IMPORTANCE OF CLEAN, FILTERED WATER

## Morning Shower Sanctuary: Clean Water, Cold Shock, & Complete Reset

Your shower should be more than a daily hygiene routine; it can be one of the most effective habit-stacking opportunities to elevate your health, beauty, and mindset before the day begins. I call it my *morning sanctuary*, a daily ritual of self-love and restoration that primes my mind and body for optimal performance.

**First and foremost—water quality matters.** Using a high-quality shower water filter is critical for protecting the skin's microbiome and moisture barrier. Chlorine, heavy metals, and volatile organic compounds (VOCs) commonly found in municipal tap water can damage the skin's lipid layer, disrupt pH, and even accelerate aging through oxidative stress. Filtered water, on the other hand, allows your skin and hair to retain natural oils and integrity, helping reduce inflammation, irritation, and dryness. It's foundational to what I call the SUPERWELL Glow.

**Then comes the contrast therapy magic.** I finish my shower with a 60–90 second cold rinse to tap into the benefits of cold water exposure. Cold showers constrict blood vessels, enhance lymphatic drainage, stimulate brown fat activation, and shift your nervous system into a state of calm alertness by activating the parasympathetic response. This natural gear shift from heightened activation into calm regulation is one of the most powerful tools you can use to train resilience and reduce systemic inflammation. Bonus: Cold water also closes the hair cuticle for extra shine and strength, and tightens pores for smoother, clearer skin.

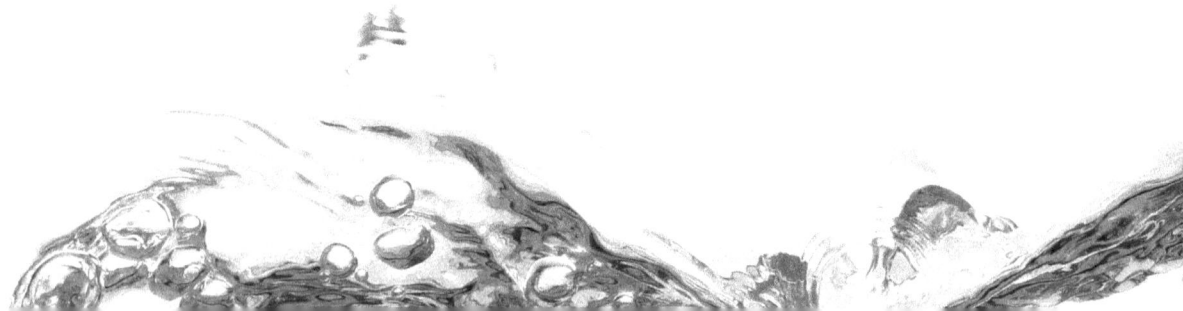

## MY HABIT STACK INSIDE THE SHOWER

I maximize every minute of this sanctuary routine. Here's how I habit stack self-care into a deeply therapeutic, multi-sensory experience.

**Aromatherapy Elevation** – I hang a eucalyptus bundle from the showerhead and diffuse stimulating essential oils like peppermint or eucalyptus to awaken the senses and clear the sinuses, or lavender and geranium for calming energy. These oils not only improve mood but have antimicrobial and anti-inflammatory properties that support respiratory and skin health.

**Deep Conditioning & Hair Healing** – I apply a deep conditioner and cover with a shower cap during the rest of my routine to trap heat and maximize absorption into the hair shaft. This is ideal for dry or chemically treated hair.

**Skin Detox + Lymphatic Boost** – While the conditioner works its magic, I use a natural body scrub to exfoliate dead skin cells, stimulate lymphatic flow, and enhance circulation, which is especially important for supporting detoxification pathways.

**Hydration Lock-In** – Post-shower, I apply a clean, nourishing body oil onto damp skin to seal in moisture, followed by a hydrating lotion to lock everything in. This double-layered technique supports the skin barrier, reduces transepidermal water loss (TEWL), and leaves skin supple and protected throughout the day.

This intentional stack of simple habits turns an everyday shower into one of the most powerful tools in my SUPERWELL routine. It's my daily reminder that self-care is not selfish; it's a necessity. When you care for yourself on a cellular level, you build a stronger, calmer, more confident you to take on the world ahead. This is always the final step in my A.M. habit stack, and the one that sets the tone for a centered, energized, and elevated day.

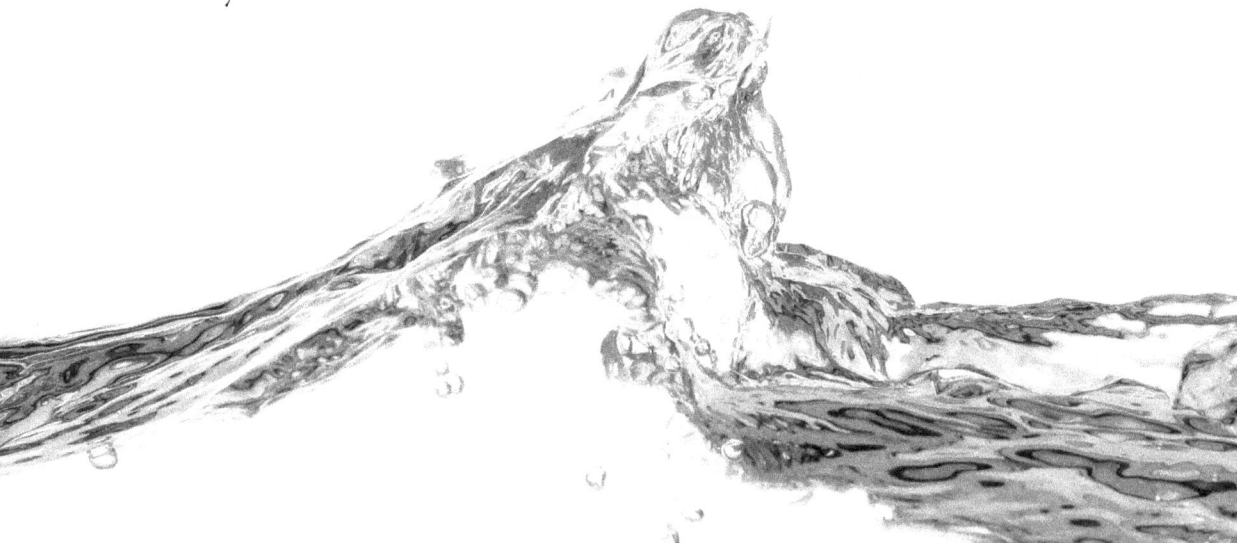

# TIME-SAVING, SOUL-FUELING TIPS
## FOR A.M. SUCCESS

Here are some of my go-to strategies to stay consistent and SUPERWELL—even on the busiest mornings.

### SET UP YOUR FUTURE SELF BEFORE BED

- Lay out your workout clothes and water bottle. No thinking required—just action.
- Measure out all your dry protein shake ingredients and mix together for a quick blend-and-go.
- Set your red light mask or meditation cushion by your bedside so it's a natural first step.

### BATCH YOUR BIOHACKS

- Turn on your infrared sauna while prepping breakfast.
- Meditate or do breathwork while on your BioMat, dry brushing, or under red light.
- Journal while sipping your gut elixir or grounding outdoors.

### DESIGN A NO-FAIL BREAKFAST STATION

- Keep all ingredients for your morning gut elixir or matcha in one organized bin to make it frictionless.
- Prep smoothie freezer packs on Sundays: individual baggies with fruit, greens, and fiber. Drop into blender; add protein and liquid; done.

## REPLACE DECISION FATIGUE WITH MICRO-INTENTIONS

- Write down your "one word" or mantra for the day on the night before, and tape it to your bathroom mirror.
- Choose your 3-2-1: 3 priorities, 2 non-negotiables, and 1 thing just for you.
- Keep a laminated list of your A.M. Habit Stack taped inside a cabinet or closet door.

## KEEP MORNING TECH-FREE AND DRAMA-FREE

- Don't open emails or texts until you have completed your stack.
- Use an old-fashioned alarm clock instead of your phone to avoid the dopamine scroll trap.
- Place your phone on airplane mode overnight and only re-engage once you have finished your breathwork, movement, or journaling.

## HABIT STACK WITH PURPOSE

- Use your cold plunge or shower time to mentally rehearse your goals.
- Listen to an audiobook or motivating podcast while walking or strength training.
- As you stretch or foam roll, list everything you are grateful for to release tension and boost your mood. It's a quick, powerful way to align body and mind with positivity.
- Set an intention while applying body oil or skincare; it's meditative and grounding.

## PREP THE ENVIRONMENT TO WIN

- Place your sneakers by the door, have your yoga mat unrolled, or place weights next to your coffee machine. Visual cues lead to action.
- Diffuse energizing essential oils like peppermint or citrus as soon as you wake up—olfactory stimulation is directly linked to memory and mood.
- Keep a warm robe or blanket by the bed to eliminate the excuse of "it's too cold to get up."

# THE SUPERWELL WAY TO 80/20 LIVING

The 80/20 principle is one of the foundations of SUPERWELL Living. It's about achieving balance, sustainability, and results without stress or restriction. It's not about perfection but consistency: making optimal choices 80% of the time while leaving 20% for enjoyment and flexibility.

## WHAT DOES 80/20 LOOK LIKE?

- 80%: Nourish your body with whole, nutrient-dense meals.
- 20%: Indulge in the foods you love, guilt-free.
- It's about living with balance while staying aligned with your goals.

## SUPERWELL EXAMPLE OF 80/20 IN A DAY

- 80%, Breakfast: Savory leftovers, protein forward, eggs, meat, avocado, and microgreens
- 80%, Lunch: Grilled chicken, quinoa, and roasted veggies
- 80%, Snack: Almonds and an apple
- 80%, Dinner: Air fryer salmon with sweet potato and steamed broccoli
- 20%, Dessert: A small bowl of homemade protein ice cream or your favorite dark chocolate treat

## FLEXIBILITY YOUR WAY

- Not into calorie counting? Think of your meals in portions: four nutrient-packed meals to every one indulgent snack or meal.
- Want a weekly approach? Dedicate one day or a few meals to favorite foods.

## WHY THE SUPERWELL METHOD LOVES 80/20

- No more deprivation: You don't have to say goodbye to the foods you love.
- Sustainable results: Consistency over extremes leads to long-term health.
- A lifestyle, not a diet: Enjoy life while staying strong, vibrant, and SUPERWELL.

## HOW TO START YOUR 80/20 LIFESTYLE:

- Focus on nutrient-rich, satisfying meals most of the time.
- Plan and enjoy your indulgences intentionally and guilt-free.
- Track what fuel feels good for you daily, weekly, or monthly.

Balance your life. Love your food.
Live SUPERWELL.

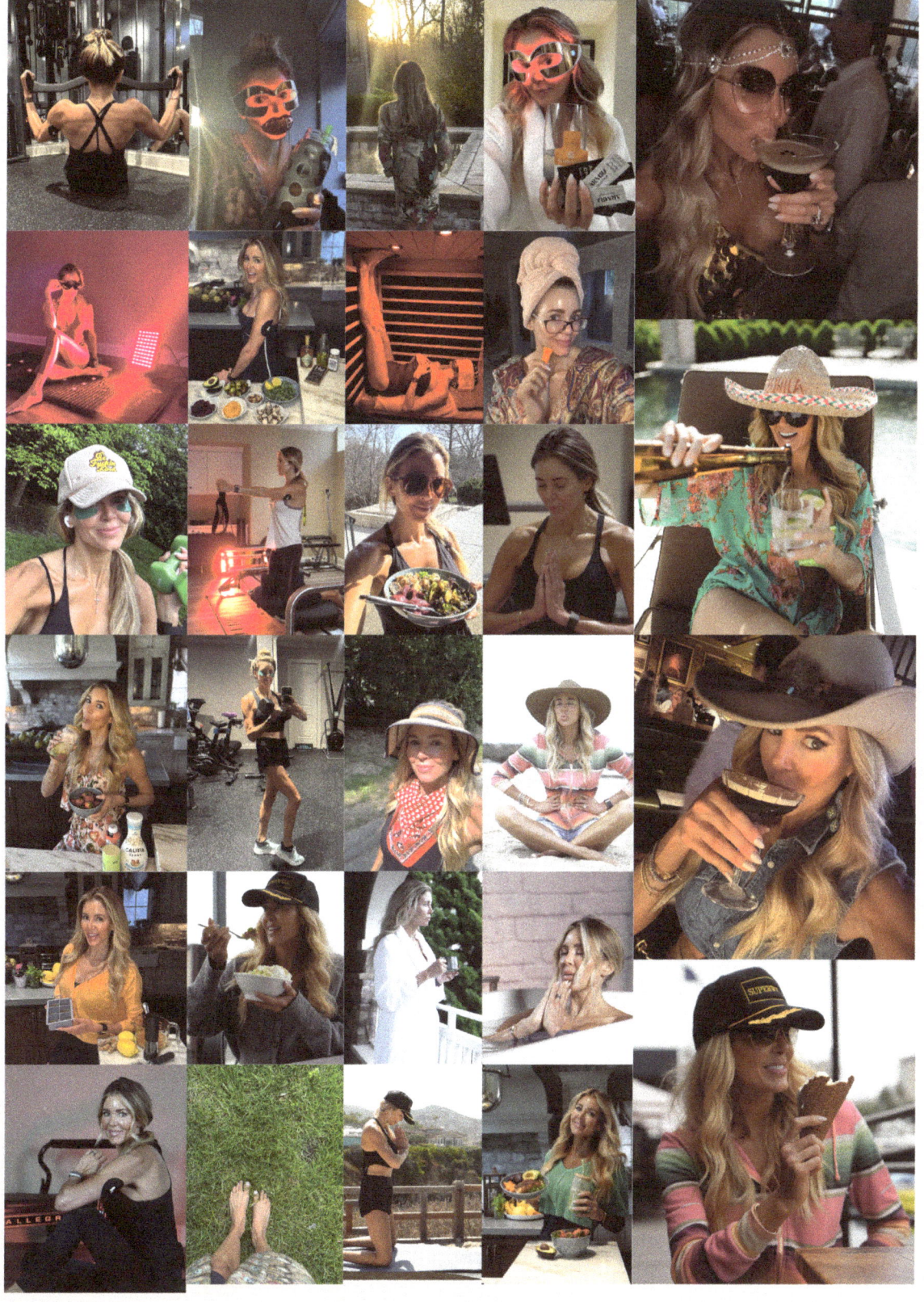

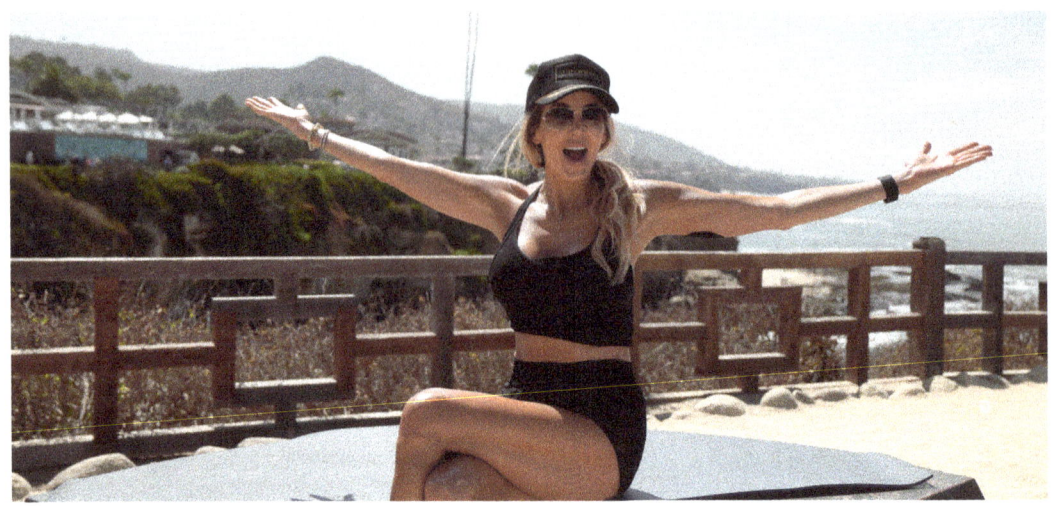

## TAKE THE LEAD:
# MASTERING YOUR MORNING MOMENTUM

Congratulations—you just gifted yourself the most important part of your day. Your morning routine is not just a list of habits; it's a daily declaration that *you* are the SUPERWELL captain of your life. When you stack your A.M. rituals with intention, you are not only boosting your energy and clarity, you are taking control of your physical, mental, and emotional trajectory. This isn't just a routine. It's your personal launchpad into a more focused, present, and purpose-driven day.

Our mornings set the tone for everything that follows. Science shows that the first 90 minutes after waking are when the brain is most impressionable—your cortisol is highest, your neuroplasticity is most active, and your decisions ripple into the rest of your day. So why not use that precious window to build habits that spark clarity, confidence, and strength?

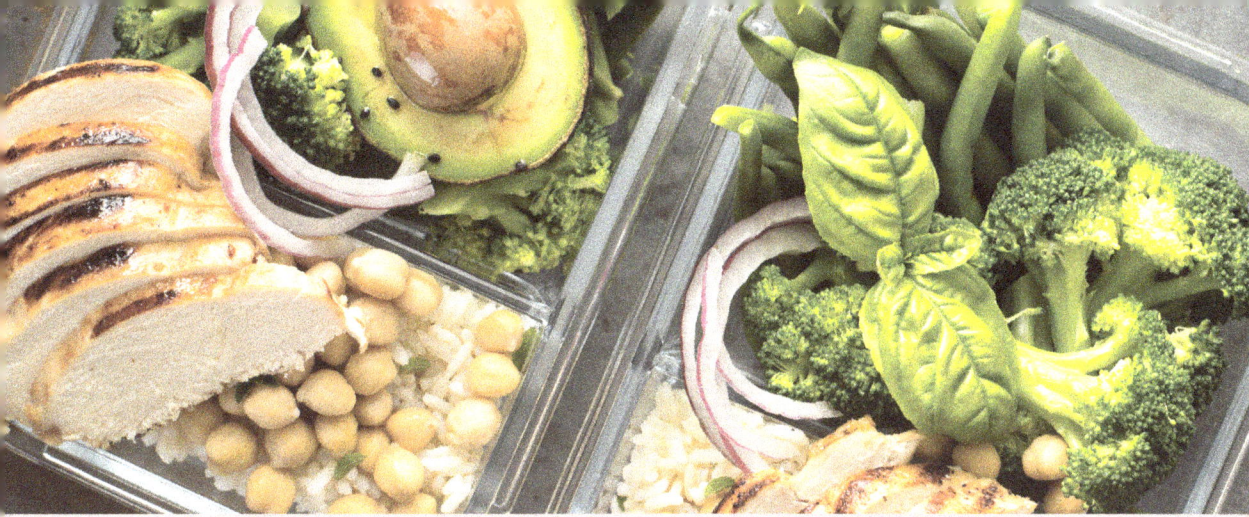

SUPERWELL

# ON-THE-GO BENTO BOX

Build-your-own travel meal designed with high-protein, high-vibe, nutrient-dense ingredients to keep you satisfied and energized in the car or at 30,000 feet. Pack it in a sectioned bento box, glass container with compartments, or reusable silicone bags.

## HOW TO BUILD YOUR BOX

Choose one to two items from Protein, one from Greens, one from Healthy Carb, one from Crunchy Snack or Nut, and one from Treats. Optional: Add a gut elixir or herbal tea bag to sip on during the flight!

## 1. PROTEIN POWER: PICK 1-2

Pack 4–6 ounces total to keep blood sugar balanced and hunger at bay.

- Grilled chicken breast, cubed or sliced, or ground chicken
- Turkey meatballs (gluten-free)
- Soft-boiled or hard-boiled eggs, halved or whole
- Sliced or ground grass-fed steak

- Smoked salmon or turkey
- Mini frittata cups (egg + veggie muffins)
- Chickpea salad (no mayo—try lemon, herbs, and olive oil)
- Baked tofu or tempeh strips

## 2. GREENS & FRESHNESS: PICK 1

Choose hydrating, alkaline greens that travel well.

- Microgreens (high in phytonutrients + fiber)
- Arugula or baby spinach
- Shredded cabbage or carrot slaw
- Sliced cucumbers or sugar snap peas
- Roasted or raw zucchini slices or roasted Brussels sprouts
- Steamed broccoli or asparagus spears

## 3. HEALTHY CARB BOOST: PICK 1

Healthy carbs add fiber, minerals, and sustained energy.

- Roasted sweet potato cubes
- Quinoa or wild rice
- Roasted chickpeas
- Hummus + veggie sticks
- Beet wedges or roasted carrots
- Grain-free crackers (like almond flour or flax crackers)

## 4. CRUNCHY SNACK OR NUT: PICK 1

Add crunch and satisfaction.

- Roasted almonds or walnuts
- Pistachios or cashews
- Toasted pumpkin seeds
- Everything bagel-seasoned roasted edamame
- Seaweed snacks
- Zen Basil seeds

## 5. THE SUPERWELL SWEET TREAT: PICK 1 SMALL PORTION

Finish with some 20%.

- 1–2 squares of 85%+ dark chocolate
- A date stuffed with almond butter + sea salt
- Dark chocolate-covered almonds (just a few!)
- Homemade protein ball
- Cacao nibs + coconut flakes combo

## EXTRA BONUS ITEMS

- Herbal tea bag (like ginger, peppermint, or chamomile), and ask for hot water on board
- Mini bottle of liquid chlorophyll or trace minerals to add to water
- A slice of lemon or lime for your water bottle

## HOW TO PACK IT LIKE A PRO

- Use silicone muffin liners or tiny containers to separate sauces, nuts, or sweet treats
- Bring a reusable bamboo fork + napkin
- Hydrate before boarding—and eat your protein + fiber first to help regulate glucose if you *do* decide to indulge in in-flight extras

## LAUREN'S GO-TO SUPERWELL COMBO

- Cubed grilled chicken + 2 hard-boiled eggs
- Handful of microgreens + arugula
- Roasted sweet potatoes
- Pumpkin seeds or toasted mixed nuts
- A square of Hu Kitchen dark chocolate with sea salt
- Peppermint tea bag for post-meal bloat control

# SUPERWELL PRO
# TRAVEL ELIXIR HACKS

Pre-pack ingredients in your empty water bottle before security. After security, buy water (or ask for hot water at a Starbucks or airport coffee shop) and mix it up for an instant wellness boost—right from your seat.

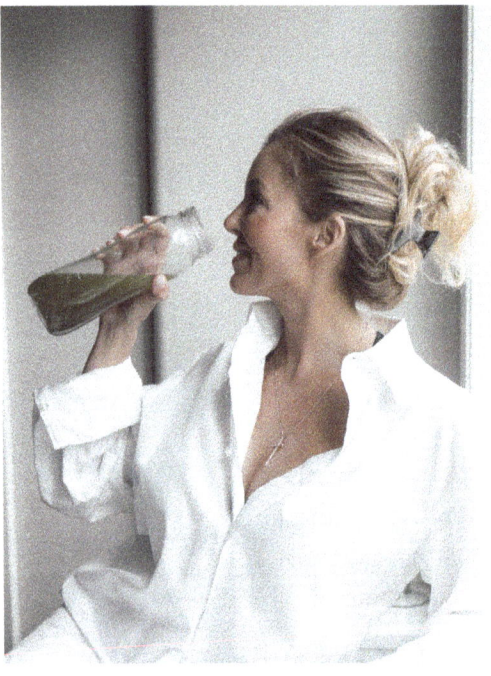

### 1. GUT RESET TRAVEL ELIXIR (FOR DIGESTION + ENERGY BOOST)

**Before security (add to empty bottle):**
- 1 tablespoon super greens powder
- 1 tablespoon apple cider vinegar powder or concentrate (or liquid in travel-safe dropper)
- Juice of 1/2 lemon or 1 tablespoon powdered lemon juice

**After security:**
- Add cold water, shake, and sip on the plane.

**Why it works:** Helps digestion, alkalizes the body, balances pH, and supports gut health while flying.

## 2. SUPERWELL BLOAT-BE-GONE ELIXIR

For de-puffing, digestion, and inflammation control mid-flight.

**Before security:**
Add the fresh or powdered ingredients to your empty glass or stainless steel bottle.

**After security:**
Add hot water (ask at a coffee counter or on the plane), let steep for 5–10 minutes, swirl or stir, and sip slowly throughout the flight.

### INGREDIENTS (CHOOSE YOUR PREP STYLE)

*Fresh Version*
(Lauren's Personal Preference)

- 1-inch piece fresh ginger, peeled + grated or thinly sliced
- 1-inch piece fresh turmeric, peeled + grated or thinly sliced
- Pinch of black pepper (enhances turmeric absorption)
- Pinch of Himalayan sea salt (for trace minerals and hydration, optional)

*Powdered Version*
(For Convenience/Travel Packs)

- 1 teaspoon ginger powder
- 1 teaspoon turmeric powder
- Pinch of black pepper
- Pinch of Himalayan sea salt (optional)

### WHY IT'S SUPERWELL APPROVED

- ✔ **Ginger** reduces bloating, supports digestion, and calms nausea.
- ✔ **Turmeric** fights inflammation and supports the liver.
- ✔ **Black pepper** boosts the bioavailability of curcumin in turmeric.
- ✔ **Himalayan salt** restores electrolyte balance after travel dehydration.

**PRO TIPS**
If you prefer a smoother texture, use a portable strainer or bring a few cheesecloth tea bags to steep and remove the fresh-grated roots after infusing.

## SUPERWELL

# GREENS & GLOW-UPS

## SUPERWELL MASON JAR SALAD BAR

A build-your-own, prep-friendly concept with layer-by-layer guidance so you can customize your own nutrient-dense, travel-ready SUPERWELL meals in a jar.

### How to Build Your SUPERWELL Salad Jar

Layer ingredients in this exact order to keep everything fresh, crisp, and delicious. Use a 24-ounce wide-mouth mason jar for the perfect fit.

1. Dressing (2–3 tablespoons)
2. Hearty veggies (to marinate in dressing)
3. Proteins
4. Grains or healthy carbs
5. Light veggies + greens
6. Toppings (for crunch and fun)

### 1. DRESSING (2–3 TABLESPOONS)

- Lemon-tahini dressing
- Apple cider vinaigrette
- Miso-ginger dressing
- Olive oil + balsamic + sea salt

### 2. HEARTY VEGGIES (1/4–1/2 CUP)

These sit in the dressing and soak up flavor.

- Cherry tomatoes
- Diced cucumbers
- Shredded carrots
- Roasted beets or Brussels sprouts (my favorite)
- Bell peppers
- Roasted sweet potatoes
- Steamed broccoli or cauliflower

### 3. PROTEINS (1/4–1/2 CUP)

- Grilled or ground chicken, beef, or bison
- Hard-boiled eggs
- Wild-caught tuna or salmon
- Black beans or lentils
- Marinated tofu or tempeh
- Falafel
- Turkey meatballs
- Quinoa + edamame combo

### 4. GRAINS OR HEALTHY CARBS (1/4–1/2 CUP)

- Cooked quinoa
- Wild rice
- Farro
- Roasted sweet potato cubes
- Chickpeas
- Brown rice
- Spiralized zucchini or carrot noodles

### 5. GREENS & LIGHT VEGGIES (1 CUP)

These go near the top to stay crisp until you shake up the jar.

- Baby spinach
- Arugula
- Romaine
- Kale (massage with olive oil + lemon, if using)
- Mixed greens
- Shredded cabbage
- Microgreens

### 6. TOPPINGS (1–2 TABLESPOONS)

- Toasted pumpkin seeds or sunflower seeds
- Chopped walnuts, almonds, or cashews, or a mix of all
- Crumbled goat cheese or feta
- Zen Basil, chia, or flax seeds (dry for crunch)
- Hemp seeds
- Pickled onions
- Sauerkraut or kimchi
- Fresh herbs (parsley, dill, basil)

**TO SERVE:** When ready to eat, give your mason jar a good shake (or pour into a bowl), mix thoroughly to coat all the layers in dressing, and enjoy!

## SUPERWELL BOWL
*Combo Inspiration*

### Gut Glow Jar
ACV vinaigrette, cucumbers, lentils, sweet potato, kale, sauerkraut, hemp seeds

### Mediterranean Mood Jar
Olive oil + lemon, cherry tomatoes, tuna, farro, arugula, olives + feta + parsley

### Taco Tuesday Jar
Cilantro-lime dressing, black beans, grilled chicken, corn + rice, romaine, crushed plantain chips

### Asian Zen Jar
Miso-ginger dressing, shredded carrots, edamame, brown rice, cabbage mix, sesame seeds + soaked Zen Basil seeds

## SUPERWELL THAI QUINOA SALAD

Bright, balanced, and bursting with texture, this Thai-inspired quinoa salad is the perfect fusion of vibrant vegetables, plant protein, and a tangy-sweet dressing that fuels your body and supports digestion. It's light enough for lunch, hearty enough for dinner, and nutrient-dense enough to keep your energy steady all day. Rich in fiber, antioxidants, and essential amino acids, this dish supports gut health, hormone balance, and sustained satiety.

- 5 large carrots, peeled and roll-cut
- 1 tablespoon olive oil (for roasting carrots)
- Sea salt to taste
- 3 cups cooked quinoa (plain or multicolored)
- 1 bunch of green onions, sliced thin
- 1 cup shelled edamame (optional for extra protein and fiber)
- 1/4 cup coconut aminos (gluten-free soy sauce alternative)
- 1 tablespoon honey or maple syrup
- 1/4 teaspoon garlic powder

**SUPERWELL PROTEIN ADD-ON SUGGESTIONS:**

- Grilled chicken breast
- Air fryer salmon
- Sesame-marinated tofu
- Seared shrimp
- Sliced flank steak

1. Preheat oven to 400°F. To roll-cut the carrots, hold your knife at an angle to the carrot and slice through. Roll the carrot so the new slice will not be parallel with the last cut, and slice again. Cut all the carrots in this way. Toss sliced carrots with olive oil and a pinch of sea salt.
2. Spread carrots in a single layer on a parchment-lined sheet pan and roast for 20 minutes or until fork-tender.
3. In a large mixing bowl, combine cooked quinoa, roasted carrots, green onions, edamame, coconut aminos, honey, garlic powder, and a pinch of sea salt.
4. Toss well until all ingredients are evenly distributed and coated in dressing.
5. Taste and adjust seasoning as needed.
6. Add protein, if desired.

### WHY IT'S SUPERWELL APPROVED

- ✔ **Blood Sugar Stability** – Quinoa is a complete protein and complex carb, which supports balanced blood sugar and sustained energy throughout the day—no spike, no crash.
- ✔ **Anti-Inflammatory Powerhouse** – This salad is rich in antioxidants from carrots and green onions, and the addition of coconut aminos provides a gut-friendly, anti-inflammatory alternative to soy sauce.
- ✔ **Protein-Rich & Customizable** – With edamame and quinoa as a plant-based protein base, plus the option to add clean proteins like salmon or grilled chicken, this dish promotes hormone balance, muscle recovery, and satiety.

## SUPERWELL NUTTY FALL KALE SALAD

Earthy, sweet, and surprisingly addictive, this is the kind of kale salad that turns skeptics into believers! Packed with antioxidant-rich greens, crunchy raw nuts, and a touch of maple for balance, it's a grounding, anti-inflammatory powerhouse. The apple cider vinegar supports digestion, while the nuts provide healthy fats to stabilize blood sugar and fuel brain health.

- 2 large bunches of lacinato or curly kale, deveined and shredded
- 1 tablespoon apple cider vinegar
- 1 tablespoon lemon juice, plus more as needed
- 2 tablespoons maple syrup
- 1/4 cup olive oil
- 1/3 cup grated parmesan cheese (sub nutritional yeast for dairy-free)
- 1 teaspoon coarse sea salt, plus more as needed
- 1/2 cup golden raisins
- 1 medium green apple, diced
- 1/2 cup raw walnuts, roughly chopped
- 1/2 cup raw pistachios, roughly chopped

1. In a large bowl, drizzle shredded kale with apple cider vinegar, lemon juice, maple syrup, and olive oil.
2. Add grated parmesan or nutritional yeast and sea salt. Massage the dressing into the kale using clean hands for about 1–2 minutes until the leaves darken and soften.
3. Add raisins, apple, walnuts, and pistachios. Toss gently until well combined.
4. Adjust seasoning with more lemon or sea salt to taste.

**SUPERWELL PROTEIN ADD-ON SUGGESTIONS:**

Warm grilled salmon fillet
Grilled chicken
Sliced roasted turkey breast
Hard-boiled eggs
Lentils or chickpeas for a plant-based option

### WHY IT'S SUPERWELL APPROVED

✓ **Hormone & Brain Health** – Walnuts and pistachios provide omega-3s and essential fatty acids that support hormone production and brain function.

✓ **Detox & Digestion Support** – Apple cider vinegar and lemon juice enhance digestion and support the body's natural detoxification pathways, especially when paired with dark leafy greens.

✓ **Blood Sugar Balance with Flavor** – The maple syrup, raisins, and apple offer natural sweetness paired with healthy fats and fiber, keeping insulin levels in check while still satisfying your palate.

## PROTEIN PUNCH CHICKEN SALAD
# Avocado Cups

Think of this as your protein-packed lunch upgrade. Creamy avocado meets crunchy chicken salad in this anti-inflammatory, hormone-supportive, and flavor-forward recipe that satisfies on every level. Great for post-workout or midday fuel.

- 2 ripe avocados, halved and pitted
- 2 cups diced grilled chicken (or rotisserie-style for ease)
- 1/4 cup finely diced red onion
- 1/4 cup finely diced celery
- 3 tablespoons Greek yogurt (organic, full-fat or low-fat)
- 1-1/2 teaspoons Dijon mustard
- 1 tablespoon avocado oil mayo
- Juice of 1 lemon (for brightness + to preserve avocado)
- Salt, to taste
- Cracked black pepper, to taste
- 2 tablespoons roasted sunflower seeds
- 1 large handful of microgreens
- Everything bagel seasoning (for extra crunch + flavor)
- Your favorite hot sauce or chili flakes for a spicy kick (optional)
- Lemon wedges

1. Scoop out a small portion of the center of the avocado halves to create a bit more room for the filling. Save for another recipe (or blend into your dressing!).

2. In a mixing bowl, combine the diced chicken, red onion, celery, Greek yogurt, mustard, mayo, lemon juice, and salt and pepper. Mix well.

3. Fold in sunflower seeds or other favorite roasted nuts for extra crunch.

4. Arrange a small bed of microgreens on each plate or serving dish. Nestle your avocado halves on top of the greens.

5. Spoon the chicken salad generously into each avocado half.

6. Sprinkle with everything bagel seasoning and drizzle with your favorite hot sauce, if desired.

7. Serve immediately with a fork and a side of lemon wedge for a final squeeze of fresh.

## WHY IT'S SUPERWELL APPROVED

✔ Protein-forward from chicken, yogurt, and seeds

✔ Healthy fats from avocado and sunflower seeds

✔ Anti-inflammatory from lemon, herbs, and microgreens

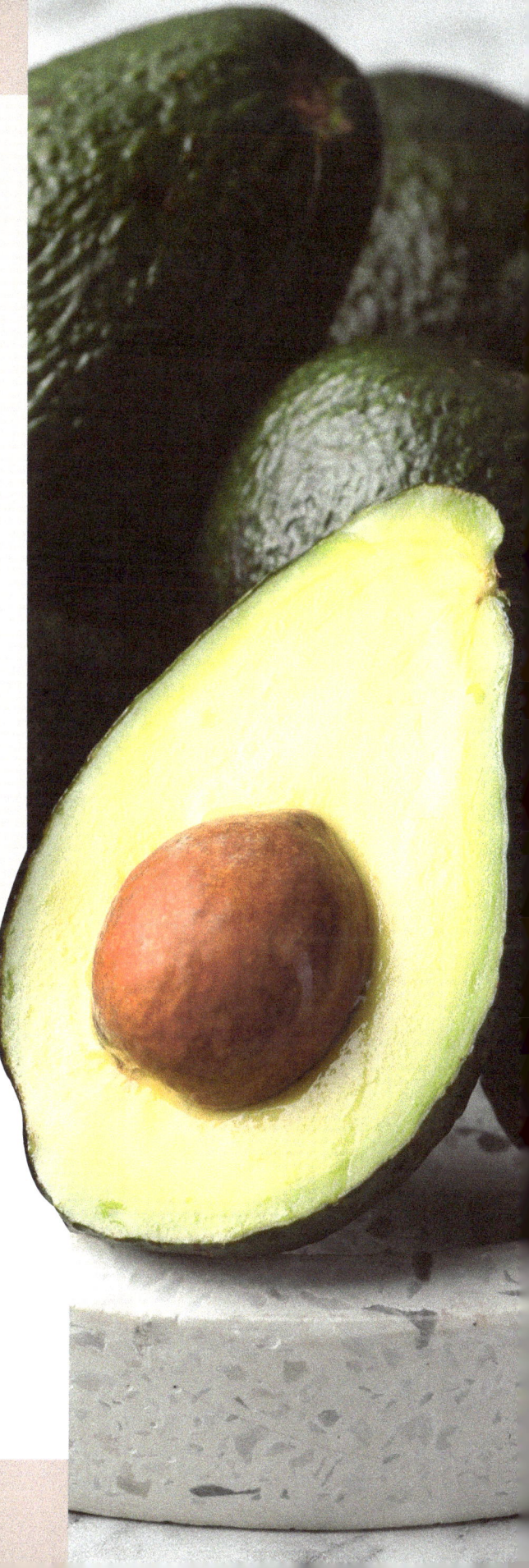

# SUPERWELL SOUPS

## SUPERWELL DETOX GLOW SOUP

This is not your average soup; it's a glow-up in a bowl! Loaded with detoxifying veggies, anti-inflammatory spices, and gut-loving broth, this vibrant blend supports digestion, skin health, and natural detox without sacrificing taste. Zucchini adds fiber and hydration; spinach or dino kale adds detoxifying chlorophyll and magnesium; lemons add brightness and skin-clearing vitamin C; and ginger is anti-inflammatory.

**YIELD: 4–6 SERVINGS**

- 1 cup organic sweet potatoes, peeled and cubed
- 1 cup organic beets, peeled and cubed
- 1 cup chopped zucchini
- 2–3 cups low-sodium beef or chicken bone broth, plus more as needed for desired consistency
- 1 cup baby spinach or chopped dino kale
- 1 (15-ounce) can organic chickpeas, drained and rinsed
- 2 cloves garlic, minced
- 2 tablespoons fresh grated ginger
- 1/2 teaspoon ground turmeric
- 1/4 cup tahini
- Juice of 2 lemons
- 1 tablespoon nutritional yeast
- 1 teaspoon sea salt, more to taste
- 2 tablespoons extra-virgin olive oil (optional)

1. In a medium pot, combine sweet potatoes, beets, zucchini, and broth. Bring to a boil, then reduce heat and simmer for 15–20 minutes until all veggies are fork-tender.
2. Add spinach or kale during the final 3–5 minutes of cooking. Let wilt slightly.
3. Let the mixture cool slightly, then transfer to a high-speed blender.
4. Add chickpeas, garlic, ginger, turmeric, tahini, lemon juice, and nutritional yeast.
5. Blend until smooth and creamy, adjusting broth for desired thickness.
6. Drizzle in olive oil while blending (optional, for a richer flavor).
7. Taste and adjust seasoning. Chill for 1–2 hours for a refreshing detox soup, or enjoy it warm!

*Optional Garnishes:*

A swirl of plain coconut yogurt

Sprinkle of hemp seeds or pumpkin seeds

Chopped parsley or cilantro

Microgreens

Cracked black pepper

Swirl of olive oil

## WHY IT'S SUPERWELL APPROVED

✔ Loaded with antioxidants for glowing skin
✔ Naturally detoxifying with beets, greens, and lemon
✔ Gut-friendly fiber and plant-based protein
✔ Anti-inflammatory from garlic, ginger, and turmeric

## SUPERWELL VEGGIE
# *Miso Soup*

Calming, mineral-rich, and immune-supportive, this veggie-packed miso soup is your answer to fast nourishment with deep impact. With gut-friendly miso, sea veggies, and warming aromatics, it's the reset your system didn't know it needed.

**YIELD: 2-3 SERVINGS**

- 3 cups filtered water
- 2 teaspoons freshly grated ginger
- 3 cloves garlic, finely grated (optional)
- 1/2 cup sliced mushrooms (shiitake or cremini work great)
- 1/2 cup shredded carrots
- 1/2 zucchini, halved and thinly sliced
- 1/2 cup baby bok choy, chopped
- 1/2 cup sliced Brussels sprouts
- 1 tablespoon dried wakame or a sheet of nori, torn
- 1/2 cup chopped spinach or kale
- 1/2 cup cubed organic soft tofu (optional, for protein)
- 3 tablespoons white or yellow miso paste (unpasteurized, if possible)
- 1 tablespoon coconut aminos (optional for depth of flavor)
- 1 teaspoon toasted sesame oil (optional for richness)
- 2 scallions, thinly sliced
- Sesame seeds or chili flakes to garnish (optional)

1. In a medium pot, bring the water, ginger, and garlic to a gentle simmer.
2. Stir in mushrooms, carrots, zucchini, bok choy, Brussels sprouts, and wakame or nori. Simmer for 5–7 minutes until veggies are just tender.
3. Add the spinach or kale and tofu cubes. Simmer another 2–3 minutes.
4. Turn off the heat. Ladle a bit of the hot broth into a small bowl and whisk in the miso paste until smooth, then stir it back into the pot. *Never boil miso to preserve its probiotics and flavor.*
5. Stir in coconut aminos and sesame oil (if using). Ladle into bowls and top with scallions, sesame seeds, or chili flakes if desired.

## WHY IT'S SUPERWELL APPROVED

✔ Miso is rich in probiotics and minerals.

✔ Sea veggies, like wakame, provide iodine + support thyroid function.

✔ Vegetables add fiber, antioxidants, and phytonutrients.

✔ Ginger + garlic support digestion and immunity.

✔ Tofu adds clean, plant-based protein.

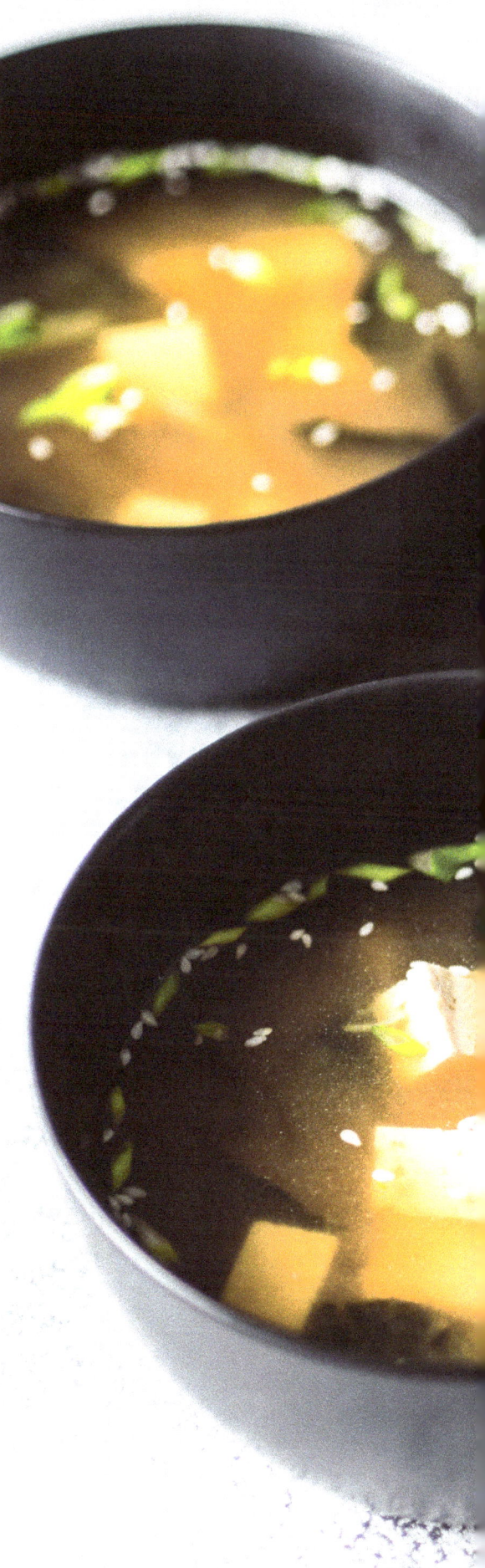

## SUPERWELL
# DRIZZLES & DIPS

These aren't just sauces; they are the secret to transforming any meal into a functional, flavor-packed experience. From creamy dressings to nutrient-rich dips, each recipe is crafted to elevate your plate with intention. Packed with healthy fats, clean ingredients, and wellness-boosting herbs and spices, these drizzles and dips are where taste meets therapeutic. Whether you're topping a salad, adding richness to a power bowl, or just need something clean and craveable to dip into, these are your go-to flavor upgrades for living SUPERWELL.

## CLASSIC GREEN GODDESS DRESSING

Herby, creamy, and totally crave-worthy.

- 1/2 cup plain Greek yogurt (or coconut yogurt for dairy-free)
- 1/4 cup packed parsley
- 2 tablespoons chopped chives
- 1 tablespoon tarragon or basil
- Juice of 1/2 or whole lemon (I love lemon, so I do the whole lemon!)
- 1 clove garlic
- 1 tablespoon olive oil or avocado oil
- Sea salt to taste
- Cracked black pepper to taste

1. Blend or process all ingredients together until smooth and creamy. Chill before serving.

## MISO-GINGER DRESSING

Savory, slightly sweet, and anti-inflammatory.

- 1 tablespoon white miso paste
- 1 tablespoon rice vinegar
- 1 teaspoon grated fresh ginger
- 1 teaspoon toasted sesame oil
- 2 tablespoons avocado or extra-virgin olive oil
- 1 teaspoon maple syrup
- 1 tablespoon water (to thin)

1. Whisk or blend all ingredients until emulsified.

## YOGURT-HERB DRIZZLE

Refreshing, cooling, and protein-boosting.

1/2 cup plain Greek yogurt

1 tablespoon lemon juice (or 2 tablespoons if you are like me and love lemon!)

1 tablespoon chopped mint or dill

1 tablespoon chopped parsley

1 small clove garlic, finely grated

Sea salt to taste

Cracked black pepper to taste

1. Stir all ingredients together in a bowl. Chill before using.

## OLIVE OIL + BALSAMIC WITH SEA SALT

A classic made SUPERWELL with clean ingredients.

2 tablespoons extra-virgin olive oil or avocado oil

1 tablespoon high-quality balsamic vinegar

Pinch of flaky sea salt

Cracked black pepper to taste

1. Shake all ingredients in a small jar or drizzle straight onto your bowl.

## COCONUT AMINOS + SESAME OIL BLEND

Umami-rich, low-glycemic, and satisfying, this blend is perfect for Asian bowls.

2 tablespoons coconut aminos

1 teaspoon toasted sesame oil

**OPTIONAL ADD-INS:**
Sprinkle sesame seeds

Green onions

Chopped water chestnuts (for extra crunch)

Red pepper flakes (for heat)

1. Mix together all ingredients, including optional add-ins. Drizzle.

## APPLE CIDER VINAIGRETTE

Simple, gut-supportive, and lightly sweetened.

3 tablespoons apple cider vinegar

1 teaspoon Dijon mustard

1 tablespoon raw honey or maple syrup

1/4 cup extra-virgin olive oil or avocado oil

Pinch of sea salt

Pinch of black pepper

1. Shake all ingredients in a jar until emulsified. Keeps well for a week in the fridge.

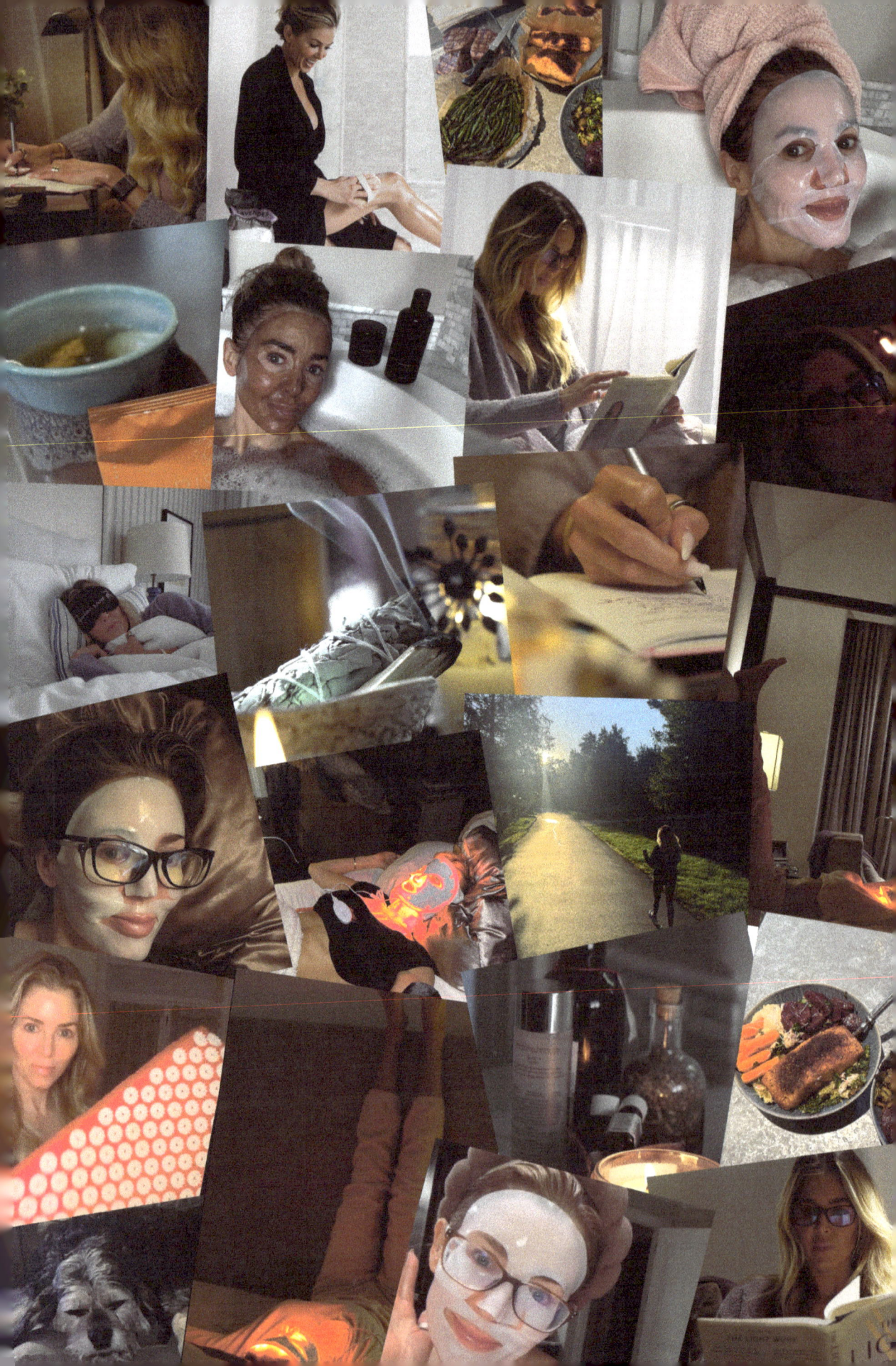

# P.M.
## HABITS

SUPERWELL

# P.M. HABIT STACKING:

## WHERE EVENING RHYTHM MEETS RESTORATIVE POWER

Your evening routine holds the key to how well your body repairs, detoxifies, and regenerates. Just like the morning sets the tone for the day, your nighttime habits set the stage for deeper sleep, balanced hormones, and cellular renewal. As the sun sets, your biology shifts, your metabolism slows, cortisol naturally lowers, and your body turns inward to heal. When you align your evening rituals with this biological blueprint, you unlock one of the most powerful yet overlooked pillars of wellness: recovery. This is your opportunity to calm the nervous system, optimize digestion, and prepare for the kind of sleep that restores you from the inside out. The goal isn't perfection—it's rhythm. And by stacking smart, science-backed habits into your evening flow, you will tap into your body's innate ability to repair, reset, and rise stronger tomorrow.

## THE POWER OF EARLY DINNERS & CIRCADIAN-ALIGNED FASTING

Finishing your last meal by 5:30 or 6:00 P.M. isn't just about convenience; it's a strategic move rooted in biology. Our digestive system is governed by the circadian rhythm, with peak efficiency occurring earlier in the day. As evening approaches, digestive enzymes, insulin sensitivity, and gut motility all begin to decline. By timing your meals to match this natural rhythm, you reduce strain on the digestive tract, optimize nutrient absorption, and promote deeper overnight repair.

Early dinners allow your body to enter an extended fast (ideally around 12 hours) before your first meal the next morning. This fasting window activates autophagy, known as the cellular "self-cleaning" process that clears out damaged cells, reduces inflammation, supports mitochondrial health, and boosts metabolic flexibility. Research shows that consistent overnight fasting improves glucose regulation, hormonal balance, and even promotes longevity by reducing oxidative stress.

## SUPERWELL TAKEAWAYS
*Why Early Dinner Is a High Impact Ritual*

### DIGESTIVE HEALTH

Giving your digestive system 3+ hours to process your final meal before sleep supports gastric emptying, reduces bloating, and minimizes the risk of acid reflux. It allows the gut lining to repair overnight, strengthening the intestinal barrier and improving microbiome balance.

### METABOLIC BOOST

Aligning your eating window with your body's natural insulin sensitivity curve (which is highest earlier in the day) supports healthier blood sugar levels. Studies show that early time-restricted eating can lead to improved fat oxidation and more efficient metabolic function.

### HORMONAL BALANCE

Melatonin (your sleep hormone) begins rising as daylight fades, while insulin sensitivity decreases. Eating late disrupts this rhythm, but an earlier dinner supports leptin and ghrelin balance—the hormones responsible for hunger and satiety—which leads to better appetite control and reduced evening cravings.

## SLEEP OPTIMIZATION

When your body isn't tasked with digesting a late meal, it can focus on repair and regeneration during sleep. Early dinner is strongly associated with improved REM and deep sleep, lower nighttime cortisol levels, and better heart rate variability (HRV).

## GUT-BRAIN RESET

The gut and brain communicate through the vagus nerve and microbial signaling. Fasting overnight enhances gut-brain communication, reduces gut inflammation, and supports production of serotonin, 90% of which is made in the gut.

## PRO TIP:
## WANT TO TAKE IT
## TO THE NEXT LEVEL?

Try closing your eating window at least 3 hours before bed and aim for a 12-hour overnight fast, even just a few days a week. This simple shift helps improve insulin sensitivity, gut repair, and cellular renewal. Pair your early dinner with a calming magnesium-rich tea, dimmed lighting, and screen-free time to signal to your body that it's time to wind down.

Remember: Small, intentional shifts in timing are not just habits; they are part of your daily blueprint for metabolic balance, longevity, and restorative sleep. You are not just eating early; you are aligning your biology with the brilliance of your internal clock.

This is more than routine, it's the rhythm of becoming SUPERWELL.

---

## SUPERWELL LIVING MEANS MAKING CHOICES TODAY
*your future self will thank you for.*

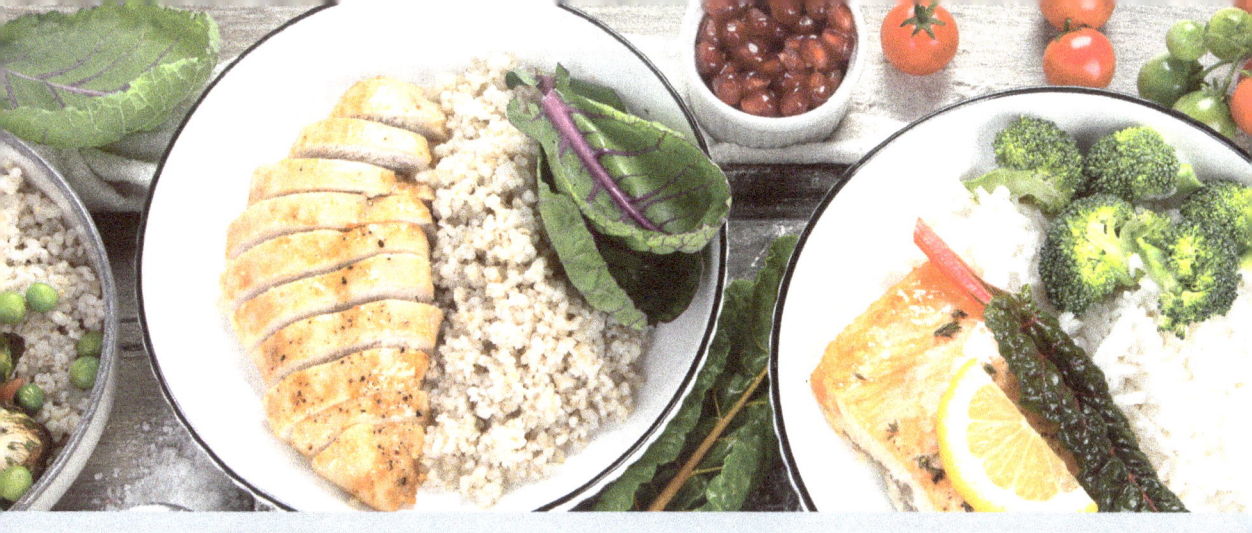

## THE SUPERWELL GLUCOSE FLOW:

# EAT SMART, STABILIZE BLOOD SUGAR, THRIVE DAILY

### WHY GLUCOSE OPTIMIZATION MATTERS

Glucose isn't just about energy; it's about mood, metabolism, hormone regulation, skin clarity, and long-term vitality. When blood sugar spikes and crashes, it creates systemic inflammation, increases aging (glycation—think toasting from the inside, which definitely doesn't help achieve that SUPERWELL glow from the inside out), impairs insulin sensitivity, disrupts hormones, and drains your energy. Learning how to eat in the right order can reduce glucose spikes by up to 73%, according to recent clinical studies.

# PRE-MEAL STRATEGY:

## SET THE STAGE FOR SUCCESS

**SUPERWELL ACV MOCKTAIL**

Starting your evening routine with an apple cider vinegar (ACV) mocktail can slow gastric emptying and blunt post-meal glucose spikes by up to 30%. Have one 5–10 minutes before eating.

1 tablespoon raw, unfiltered apple cider vinegar

8 oz filtered still or sparkling water

Squeeze of lemon or lime

Drop of organic stevia, a cinnamon stick, or even favorite berries (optional)

1. Combine all ingredients in a glass and enjoy. This helps pre-activate digestion, lowers glycemic response, and can support insulin sensitivity.

**PRO TIP** Sip your ACV mocktail with a straw to protect your tooth enamel.

# 6 SUPERWELL MOCKTAILS

## 1. SUPERWELL SPARKLER

A fresh, fizzy gut-supporting mocktail perfect for glowing skin and balanced digestion.

- 1 tablespoon apple cider vinegar
- Juice of 1/2 lemon or lime
- 1 teaspoon maple syrup or a few drops of liquid stevia (optional)
- Fruit and herbs of choice (see below)
- Crushed ice
- Sparkling water

*Fun Flavor Add-Ins:*

Fresh cucumber slices + mint

Smashed blackberries + rosemary

Blood orange slices + basil

1. Add ACV, citrus juice, and sweetener to a glass. Muddle your chosen fruit + herbs in the bottom. Add crushed ice and top with sparkling water. Stir and enjoy!

## 2. THE ZEN FIZZ

Calming, mineral-rich, and perfect before or after meals.

- 1/4 teaspoon grated fresh ginger (or 1 thin slice)
- 1 tablespoon fresh cucumber juice (or 2–3 slices of muddled cucumber)
- A few mint leaves
- 1 teaspoon lemon juice
- Pinch of Himalayan salt
- Still or sparkling water
- Crushed ice

*Optional Additions:*

1 slice jalapeño for a little heat

Sliced fennel bulb for digestive support

1. Muddle ginger, cucumber, and mint in the glass. Add lemon juice and salt. Fill with ice, top with water, and stir well.

## 3. THE GLOW-UP TONIC

Bright, citrusy, and packed with antioxidants and hydration.

- Juice of 1 grapefruit or orange
- Squeeze of lemon
- Splash of unsweetened pomegranate or cranberry juice
- Ice
- Orange or grapefruit slices
- Sparkling water
- Basil or mint sprigs

*Flavor Twists*

- Add pomegranate seeds for crunch.
- Sub blood orange for a winter version.
- Muddle fresh thyme for a savory finish.

1. Combine juices in a shaker or glass with ice. Shake or stir, pour over fresh citrus slices, and top with sparkling water and herbs.

## 4. THE DETOX GARDEN MOCKTAIL

Earthy, hydrating, and perfect for a spa day or Sunday reset.

- 1 small handful of chopped celery
- 1 inch cucumber, grated
- 1 tablespoon chopped parsley or mint
- Still water or coconut water
- Juice of 1/2–1 lime
- 1 teaspoon honey or monk fruit
- Ice

*Optional Additions:*

- Splash of aloe juice
- Zen Basil seeds (soaked and stirred in)
- Dash of cayenne for a metabolism kick

1. Blend celery, cucumber, and herbs with water. Strain if preferred. Stir in lime juice and sweetener. Serve over ice.

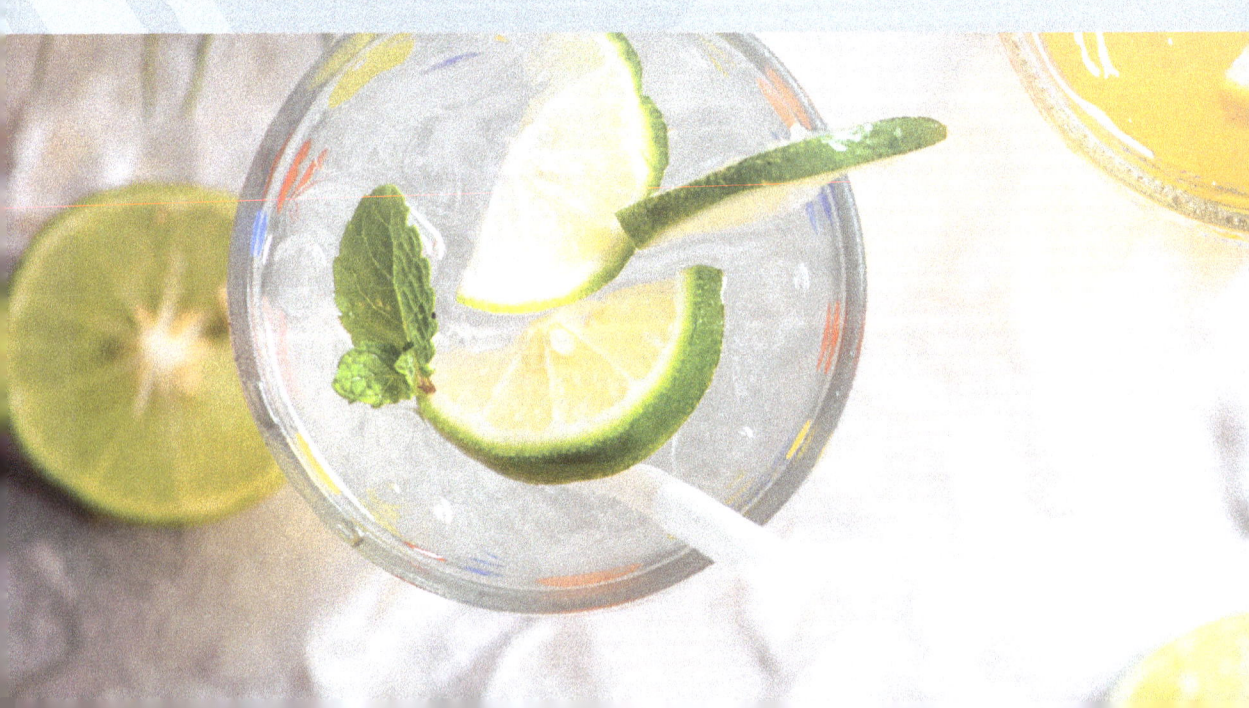

## 5. THE SUPERWELL SUNSET

This fruity, slightly tangy, and beautiful layered mocktail feels like a treat.

- 1/3 cup mango or peach puree
- 1/3 cup chilled hibiscus or berry herbal tea
- 1/3 cup sparkling water
- Juice of 1/2–1 lime, or to taste
- Edible flowers or citrus peel twist (optional, garnish)

### Flavor Twists

- Add frozen berries as ice cubes.
- Blend with ice for a frozen slushy version.
- Stir in 1 teaspoon collagen powder for a glow boost.

1. Layer mango puree at the bottom, pour tea over the back of a spoon to float on top, and finish with sparkling water + lime. Garnish if desired.

## 6. THE MINTY MELON COOLER

Refreshing, cooling, and full of electrolytes—this is great post-workout or poolside.

- 1 cup fresh watermelon or honeydew chunks
- Juice of 1/2–1 lime
- Handful of mint leaves
- Pinch of sea salt
- Ice
- Sparkling water or coconut water
- Mint sprigs (garnish)

### Optional Add-Ins:

- Cucumber slices
- Frozen grapes or kiwi cubes
- Dash of ginger

1. Blend melon, lime juice, mint, and salt into a puree. Pour over ice, top with sparkling water or coconut water, and garnish with mint sprigs.

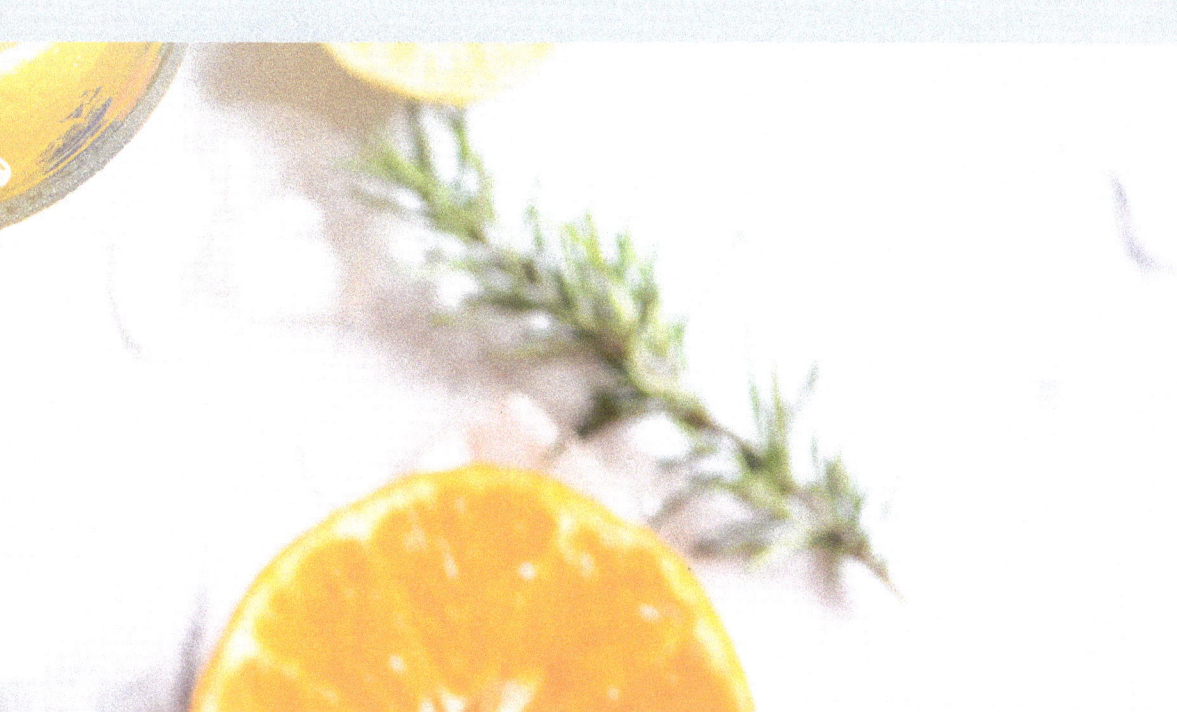

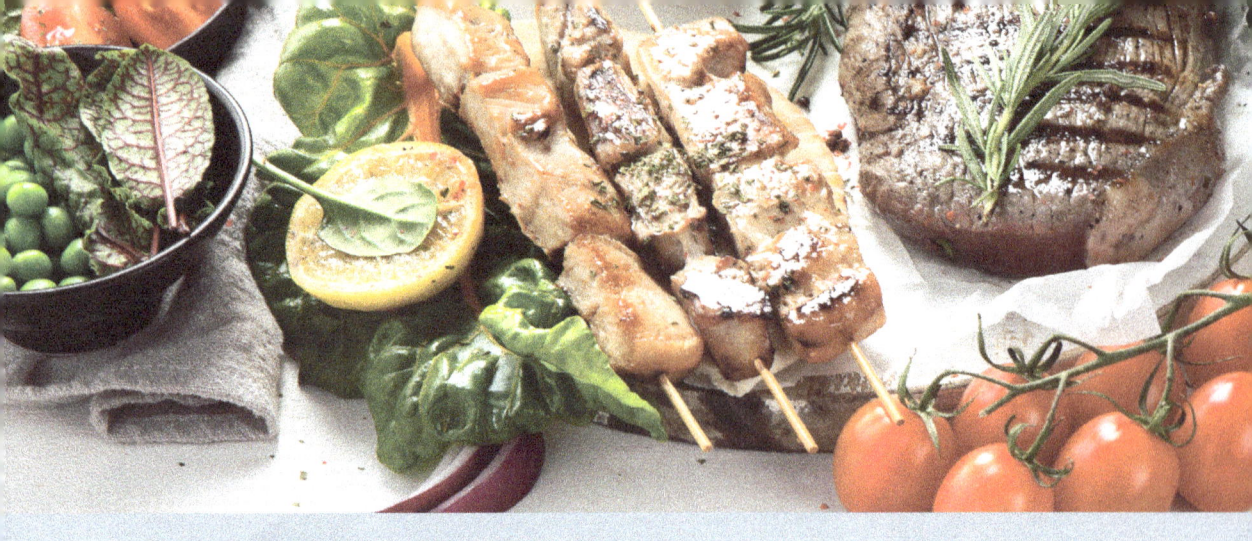

## THE ORDER MATTERS:

# HOW TO EAT YOUR MEAL LIKE A SUPERWELL SUPERSTAR

Food order matters: Begin meals with a veggie-based starter, then protein and healthy fats, and finish with smart carbs. This order can reduce glucose spikes significantly.

### 1. START WITH FIBER: LEAFY GREENS, CRUCIFEROUS VEGGIES & HERBS

Eating fiber first (think Brussels sprouts, microgreens, arugula, spinach, kale, broccoli, cauliflower, or a side salad with olive oil and lemon) creates a viscous mesh in the gut that slows down glucose absorption. This "fiber shield" delays sugar release into the bloodstream and improves satiety.

**Pro Tip:** Add apple cider vinegar or other vinegars or lemon juice to your greens for double the glucose-lowering effect. Double whammy!

## 2. NEXT UP: PROTEIN & HEALTHY FATS

Prioritize lean proteins like wild salmon, organic chicken, bison, grass-fed beef, eggs, or legumes. Pair with healthy fats like avocado, extra-virgin olive or avocado oil, nuts, and seeds. Protein and fat buffer carbohydrate absorption, support muscle synthesis, and keep hunger hormones in check (ghrelin and leptin).

## 3. *THEN* EAT YOUR CARBOHYDRATES

Whether it's sweet potatoes, brown rice, quinoa, roasted root veggies, or even sourdough bread, the key is to save them for the third part of your meal. By eating carbs last, you significantly reduce the rate of glucose entering your bloodstream.

## 4. IF YOU ARE HAVING DESSERT, MAKE IT THE FINALE

Enjoy treats *after* a balanced meal (never on an empty stomach). Add cinnamon, lean protein, or fat to slow the sugar impact (e.g., dark chocolate with peanut or almond butter). Walk for 15–20 minutes after eating to aid in postprandial glucose clearance.

## BONUS SUPERWELL TIPS FOR DAILY GLUCOSE OPTIMIZATION

**Morning Movement Matters** – A brisk walk, strength training, or a Pilates session in the morning helps activate insulin receptors and improves glucose disposal throughout the day.

**Avoid Bare-Naked Carbs** – Always pair carbohydrates with fat, fiber, or protein.

**Walk After Meals** – Just 10–20 minutes of walking can reduce your glucose spike by 22–30%.

**Don't Skip Protein at Breakfast** – Aim for 30+ grams to start your day with stable blood sugar and reduced cravings.

# "YES" FOODS TO ENJOY CLOSER TO BEDTIME

These foods support nervous system regulation, melatonin production, hormone repair, and blood sugar balance. These are the foundation for restful, restorative sleep.

## 1. TRYPTOPHAN-RICH PROTEINS (BUILD SEROTONIN & MELATONIN)

**Why:** These proteins support production of calming neurotransmitters for mood and sleep.

**Examples:**

- Organic turkey or chicken (2–4 ounces)
- Cottage cheese or Greek yogurt (if tolerated)
- Pasture-raised eggs
- Collagen peptides or bone broth protein (gentle on digestion)

## 2. MAGNESIUM & POTASSIUM-RICH FOODS (CALMING MINERALS)

**Why:** Magnesium soothes the nervous system; potassium supports muscle relaxation and sleep depth.

**Examples:**

- 1/2 banana with almond butter
- Avocado slices with sea salt
- Pumpkin seeds or sunflower seeds
- Chia or Zen Basil seeds (soaked overnight), mixed with some Greek yogurt
- Spinach sautéed in olive oil

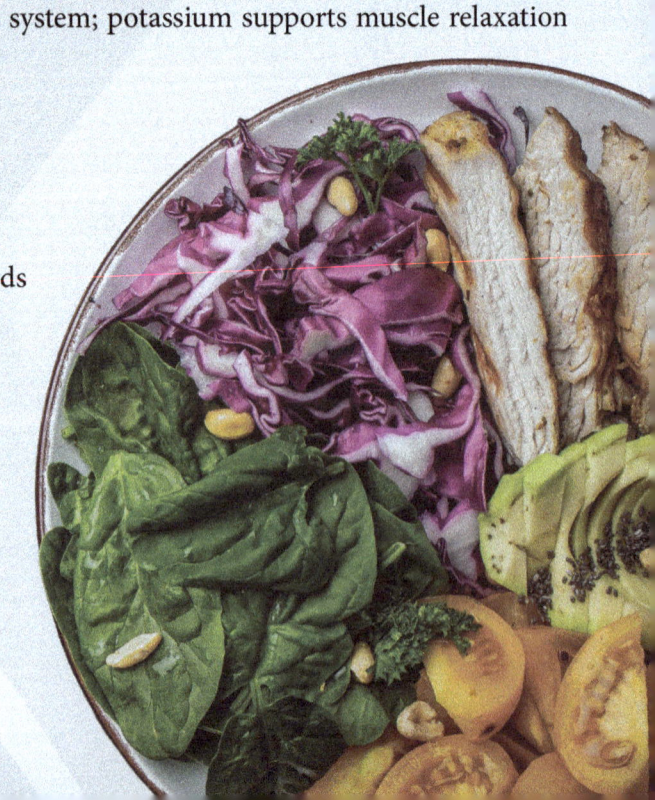

## 3. SLOW-DIGESTING CARBOHYDRATES (BALANCE BLOOD SUGAR)

**Why:** A small amount of complex carbs can help lower cortisol and promote melatonin release.

**Examples:**

- Sweet potato mash or roasted cubes
- 1/4 cup cooked oats or quinoa
- A few berries (with fat or protein), mixed with Greek yogurt
- Sliced apple with tahini or nut butter

## 4. HEALTHY FATS (FOR HORMONE AND BLOOD SUGAR STABILITY)

**Why:** Fats slow digestion, reduce blood sugar spikes, and support hormone production.

**Examples:**

- 1 tablespoon almond butter, peanut butter, sunflower butter, or coconut butter
- Handful of raw nuts (almonds, walnuts, Brazil nuts)
- Tahini or avocado drizzled with olive oil

## 5. CAFFEINE-FREE HERBAL TEAS (SLEEP SUPPORTIVE)

**Why:** Herbal infusions calm the mind, reduce cortisol, and signal the body to wind down.

**Examples:**

- Chamomile or lavender (gentle nervous system support)
- Lemon balm or passionflower (anxiolytic properties)
- Tulsi Holy Basil (cortisol regulation)
- Valerian root blends (supports sleep onset and depth)

## "NO" FOODS TO AVOID CLOSER TO BEDTIME

These foods may disrupt blood sugar balance, digestion, hormone production, and nervous system regulation, and keep you wired when your body should be resting.

### 1. SUGARY SNACKS & REFINED CARBS

**Why to Avoid:** Spikes blood sugar, then leads to a crash, triggering cortisol as your body tries to stabilize glucose levels, often resulting in mid-sleep wakeups.

**Examples:** Candy, pastries, white bread, sugary cereals, granola bars, and processed snack foods

### 2. CAFFEINE (EVEN HIDDEN SOURCES)

**Why to Avoid:** Caffeine blocks adenosine (a sleep-inducing neurotransmitter), delays melatonin release, and increases cortisol production, making it harder to fall and stay asleep.

**Examples:** Coffee, energy drinks, green/black tea, chocolate, and decaf (if sensitive)

### 3. ALCOHOL

**Why to Avoid:** Initially sedating, alcohol disrupts REM cycles and elevates cortisol as it metabolizes. This results in lighter, fragmented sleep and early wake-ups.

**Examples:** Wine, beer, cocktails, and hard seltzers

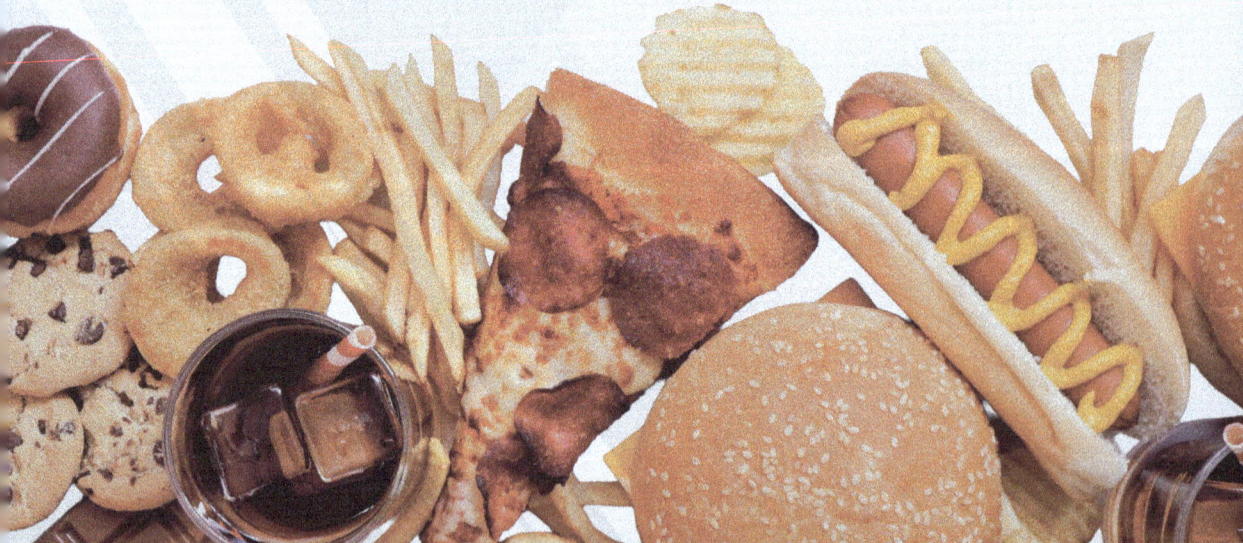

## 4. SPICY FOODS

**Why to Avoid:** Can raise internal body temperature and cause digestive irritation, which elevates cortisol and disrupts sleep onset and depth.

**Examples:** Chili flakes, hot sauce, curry, wasabi, and heavily seasoned meats

## 5. HIGH-FAT, HEAVY MEALS

**Why to Avoid:** Delays digestion and keeps the body metabolically active when it should be transitioning to rest. This also raises nighttime cortisol.

**Examples:** Fried foods, creamy pasta, loaded burgers, and rich cheese-heavy dishes

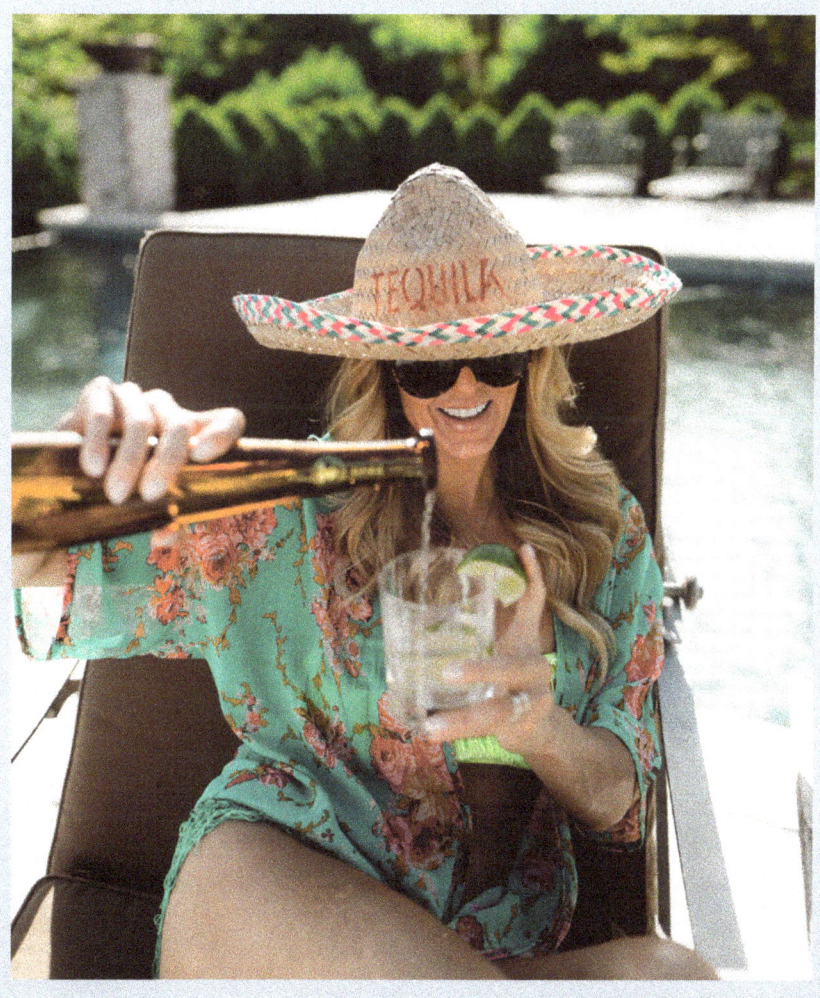

## THE BOTTOM LINE

Glucose optimization isn't about restriction, it's about *order, timing,* and *pairing*. When you stack these practices together—such as ACV before meals, fiber first, protein next, carbs last, mindful and smart sweets—you create a flow and blueprint that supports longevity, hormonal balance, stable energy, and even SUPERWELL glowing skin.

Now that's what we call eating SUPERWELL smart!

### PRO TIP:

Stack your bedtime snack with protein + fat + fiber + optional slow-digesting carbs to stabilize blood sugar and enhance overnight recovery. For example: a warm mug of magnesium-rich tea + collagen + sweet potato cube + nut butter drizzle = SUPERWELL slumber.

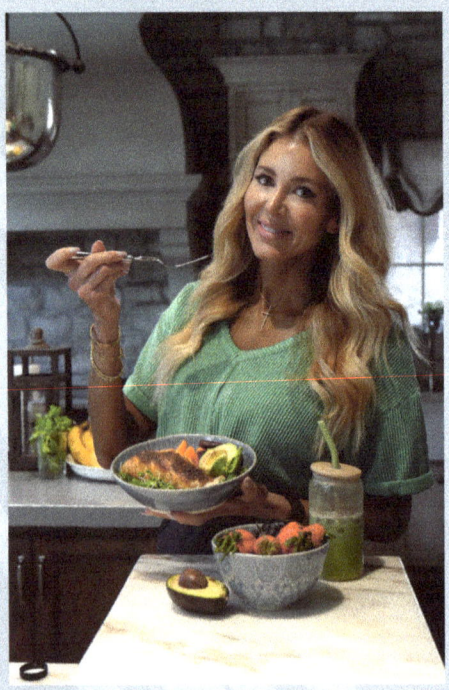
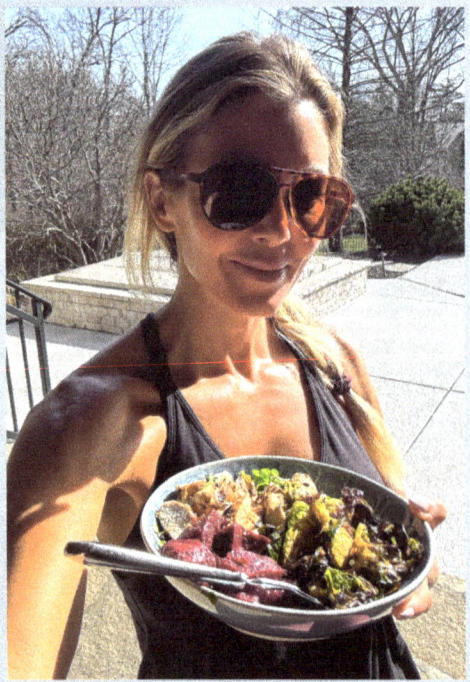

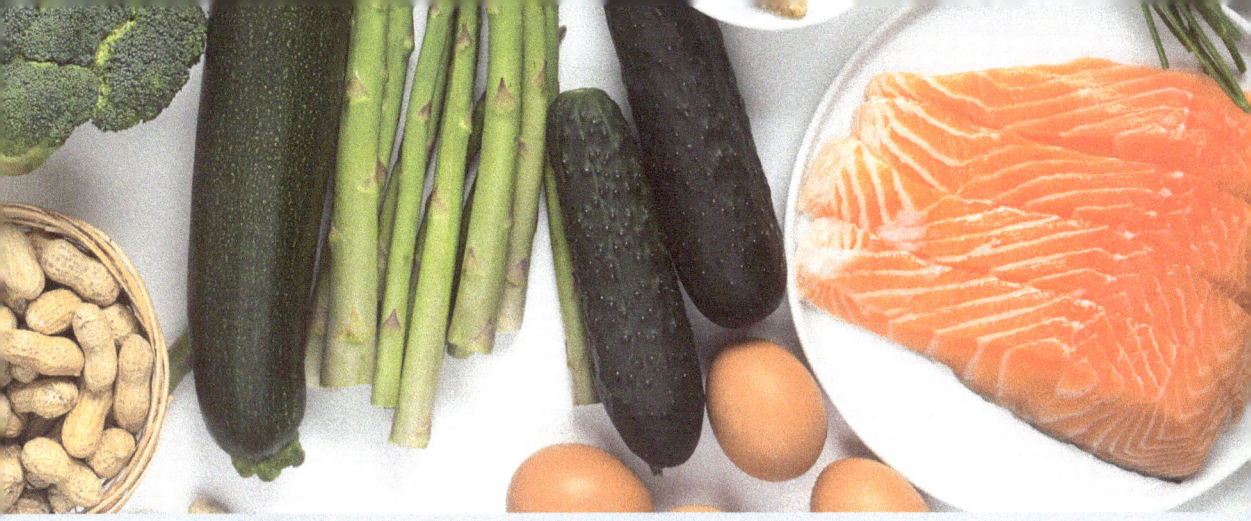

# SUPERWELL CHEAT SHEET:
# UNDERSTANDING MACROS

Macros (macronutrients) are the building blocks of a balanced diet and are key to achieving your fitness, energy, and wellness goals. They provide a deeper understanding of how food fuels your body beyond just calories. Let's break it down the SUPERWELL way!

## MACROS VS. CALORIES: WHAT'S THE DIFFERENCE?

Calories give you a total number but don't tell you where the energy is coming from (protein, carbs, or fats). You can lose weight by tracking calories, but you might lose muscle along with fat and feel fatigued if the balance is off. Macros break calories into protein, carbs, and fats, focusing on body composition (muscle vs. fat), energy, and performance. Tracking macros helps preserve muscle, optimize workouts, and maintain steady energy levels.

**WHY MACROS MATTER**
Calories = Weight change
Macros = Muscle, energy, and body composition

## PROTEIN:
## The Building Block of Life

### WHAT IS IT?
Protein is made of amino acids that repair and grow muscle, support enzymes, and aid in hormone production. It's found in meat, fish, eggs, dairy, legumes, tofu, and grains.

### WHY DO WOMEN NEED IT?
**Muscle Maintenance** – Essential for staying strong, especially as you age.

**Satiety** – Keeps you full longer, helping with weight management.

**Bone Health** – Supports collagen and bone density.

### HOW MUCH?
Aim for 1 gram per pound of goal body weight or more! Example: A 150-pound woman aiming for 135 pounds should eat 135 grams of protein per day.

### SUPERWELL PROTEIN EXAMPLES:
- 2 eggs = 13 g protein
- 100 g chicken breast = 31 g protein
- 100 g tofu = 26 g protein

## CARBOHYDRATES:
## Your Energy Source

### WHAT ARE THEY?
Carbs break down into glucose, which fuels your brain, muscles, and organs. They're found in bread, rice, pasta, fruits, vegetables, and grains.

### WHY DO WOMEN NEED THEM?
**Energy** – Carbs power workouts and recovery.
**Brain Health** – Essential for focus and cognitive function.
**Hormonal Balance** – Regulates insulin and supports menstrual health.

### HOW MUCH?
Aim for 40–60% of daily calories depending on activity level. Prioritize complex carbs (whole grains, vegetables, fruits) over refined carbs.

### SUPERWELL CARB EXAMPLES:
- 100 g sweet potato = 20 g carbs
- 1 banana = 20 g carbs
- 1 cup quinoa = 39 g carbs

## FATS:
### Essential for Hormones & Long-Term Energy

**WHAT ARE THEY?**

Fats help your body absorb vitamins, support brain function, and provide sustained energy. They're found in avocados, nuts, seeds, olive oil, and fatty fish.

**WHY DO WOMEN NEED THEM?**

**Hormonal Health** – Critical for estrogen and progesterone production.
**Skin & Hair** – Keeps your skin hydrated and your hair strong for that SUPERWELL glow!
**Energy** – Provides long-lasting fuel for low-intensity activities.

**HOW MUCH?**

Aim for 20–35% of daily calories from healthy fats. Include at least 40 grams of healthy fats per day.

**SUPERWELL FAT EXAMPLES:**
- 1/2 avocado = 15 g fat
- 1 tablespoon olive oil = 14 g fat
- 100 g salmon = 13 g fat

## MACROS MADE SIMPLE:

**Protein** – The builder (repair and muscle).
**Carbs** – The fuel (energy and recovery).
**Fats** – The supporter (hormones and brain).

Tracking macros isn't about restriction—it's about understanding what your body needs to thrive, perform, and feel SUPERWELL.

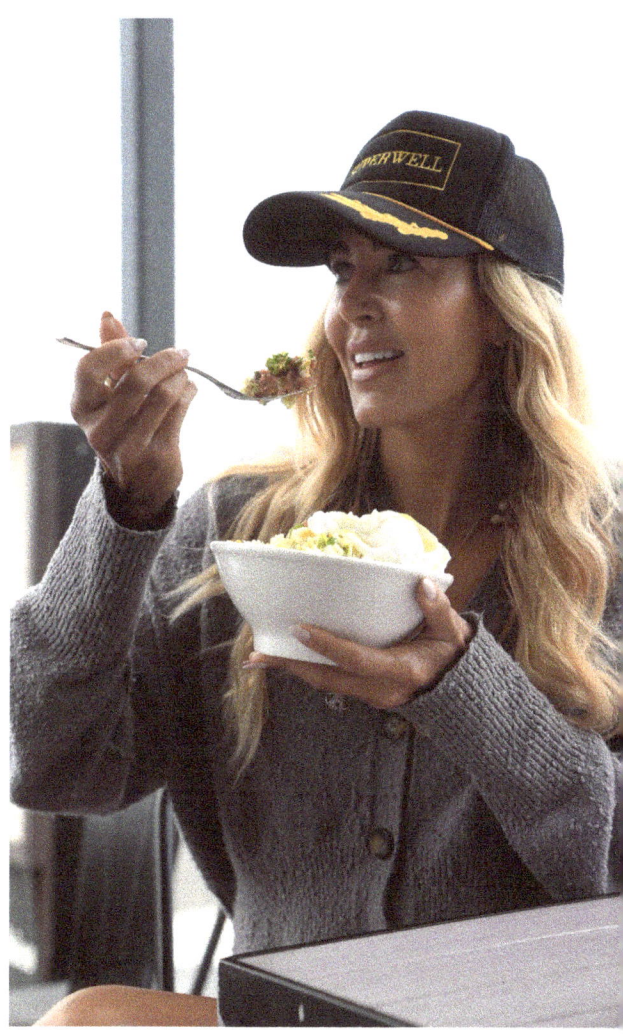

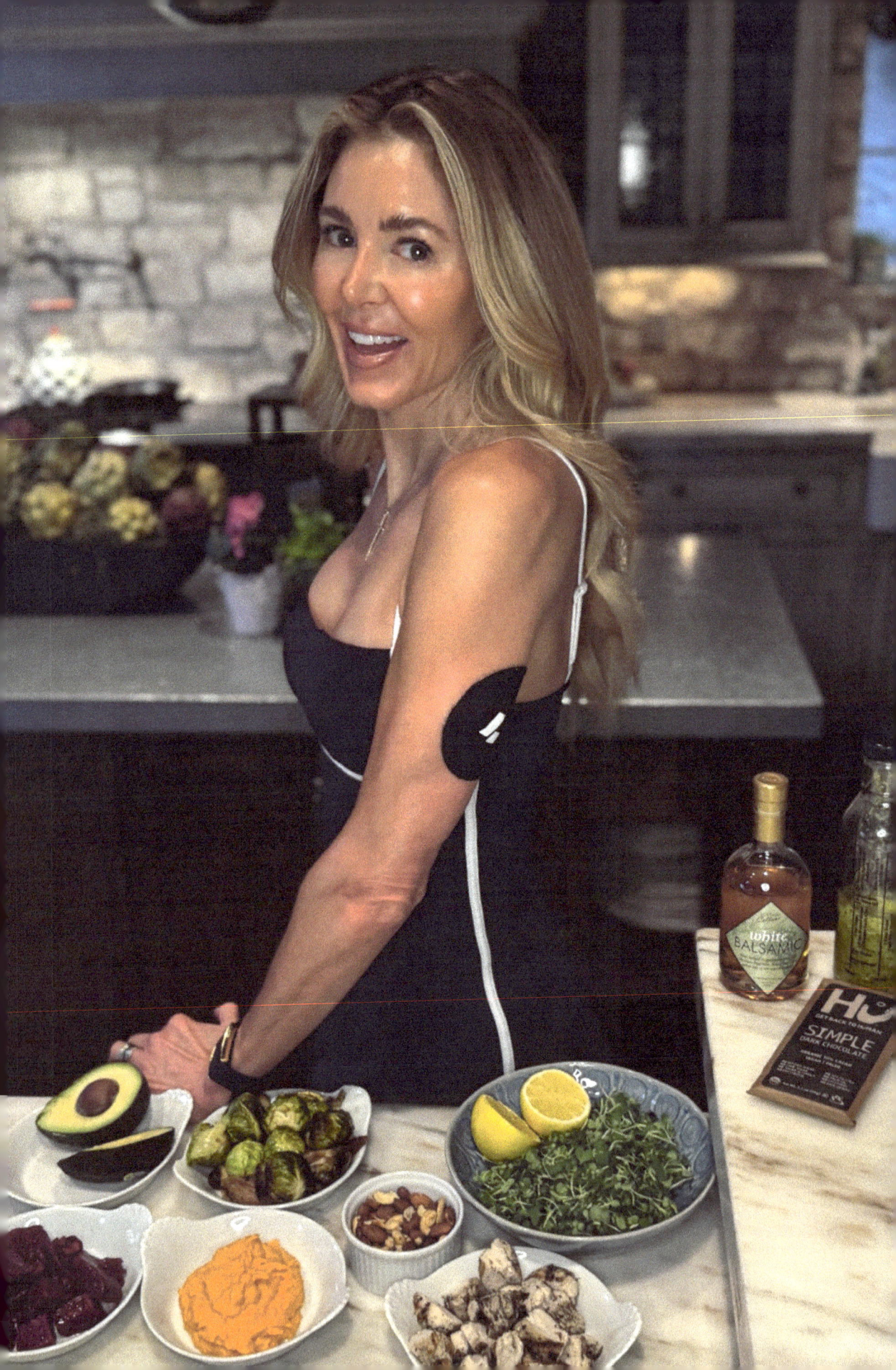

## STRONG > SKINNY:
# REDEFINING THE WHY BEHIND WHAT YOU EAT

Somewhere along the way, society taught us that eating less was a badge of honor. That shrinking ourselves was the goal. But let me be clear: I have lived through that mindset, and it nearly broke me. I was inflamed, puffy, exhausted, and my skin looked tired even though I was "doing all the right things." I wasn't fueling; I was fighting against my body.

When I finally let go of the idea that thinness equaled wellness and started nourishing my body for energy, strength, and clarity, everything changed. I stopped counting calories and started counting colors on my plate. I prioritized protein, healthy fats, hydration, minerals, and fiber; in return, my body started to show up for me in a big way.

We are not here to simply get by. We are here to feel strong, energized, and alive. That doesn't happen through restriction; it happens through intentional nourishment.

Eating to feel SUPERWELL means:

- Prioritizing blood sugar balance to avoid crashes and mood swings.
- Building lean muscle through adequate protein to support metabolism and longevity.
- Choosing whole foods that stabilize hormones and promote deep cellular repair.
- Creating meals that feed your brain, your gut, and your spirit.

Let's also not forget: Undereating is a stressor. Chronically under-fueling sends a message to your body that it's not safe, and when your body doesn't feel safe, it holds onto everything. The weight, the fatigue, the brain fog. That's not failure; that's physiology.

I want to help you flip the script and use this as your blueprint. I want you to eat like someone who has dreams to chase, a life to build, and energy to burn. I want you to eat like someone who loves their body enough to fuel it like the masterpiece it is.

So no, I don't eat to be skinny. I eat to feel focused, powerful, and capable.

And you can too.

This isn't about restriction. This is about *restoration*. This isn't about fear. It's about *fuel*. This is what it means to live SUPERWELL.

Let's stop starving and start thriving.

---

**SUPERWELL LIVING LETS YOU *rewrite the rules*, ONE MINDFUL HABIT AT A TIME.**

---

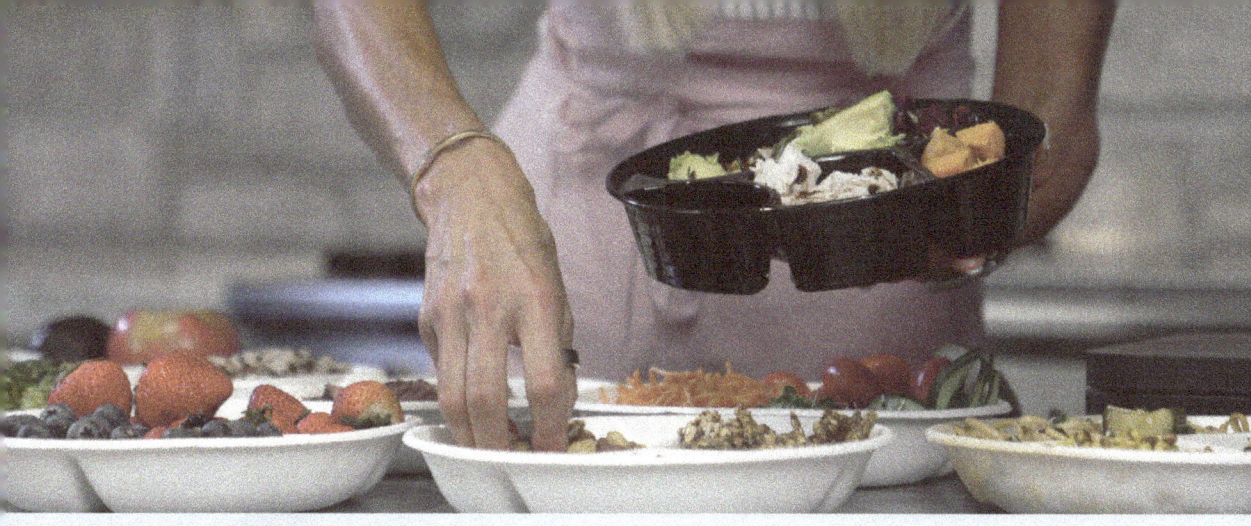

SUPERWELL

# P.M. PLATES

## SUPERWELL BUILD-YOUR-OWN POWER BOWL BAR

A fun, mix-and-match protein bowl concept featuring clean proteins, slow carbs, vibrant greens, and rainbow veggies that is designed to nourish, energize, and satisfy.

**Perfect For:**
- Family-style dinners
- Meal prep for the week
- Post-workout refuel
- "What do I feel like today?" moments

## HOW IT WORKS

Pick 1 from each category:

- Protein (for strength + satiety)
- Grain or Healthy Carb (for energy + balance)
- Greens (for volume + fiber)
- Rainbow Veggies (for antioxidants + crunch)
- Sauce or Dressing (to bring it all together)
- Toppings (for texture, flavor, and variety!)

You can prep ingredients in advance, store in separate containers, and assemble in minutes!

## 1. PICK YOUR PROTEIN

- Grilled organic chicken or steak
- Ground beef, bison, turkey, or chicken with taco spices
- Wild-caught salmon or tuna
- Hard-boiled eggs
- Marinated tofu or tempeh
- Baked falafel
- Boiled or roasted edamame
- Lemon-garlic shrimp
- Lentils or black beans

## 2. CHOOSE A GRAIN OR HEALTHY CARB

- Quinoa
- Farro
- Brown rice or wild rice
- Roasted sweet potato cubes
- Cauliflower rice (for low-carb option)
- Millet
- Soba noodles
- Chickpea pasta (cold)
- Roasted spaghetti squash

## 3. ADD YOUR GREENS

- Baby spinach
- Arugula
- Massaged kale
- Butter lettuce
- Spring mix
- Romaine
- Shredded cabbage
- Microgreens (as a garnish or base)

## 4. LOAD UP RAINBOW VEGGIES

- Red: cherry tomatoes, red bell peppers, radishes
- Orange: roasted carrots, shredded carrots, sweet potato
- Yellow: golden beets, corn, yellow bell peppers
- Green: cucumbers, Brussels sprouts, zucchini ribbons, green beans, broccoli
- Purple: red cabbage, purple cauliflower, roasted eggplant
- White: roasted cauliflower, hearts of palm, shaved fennel

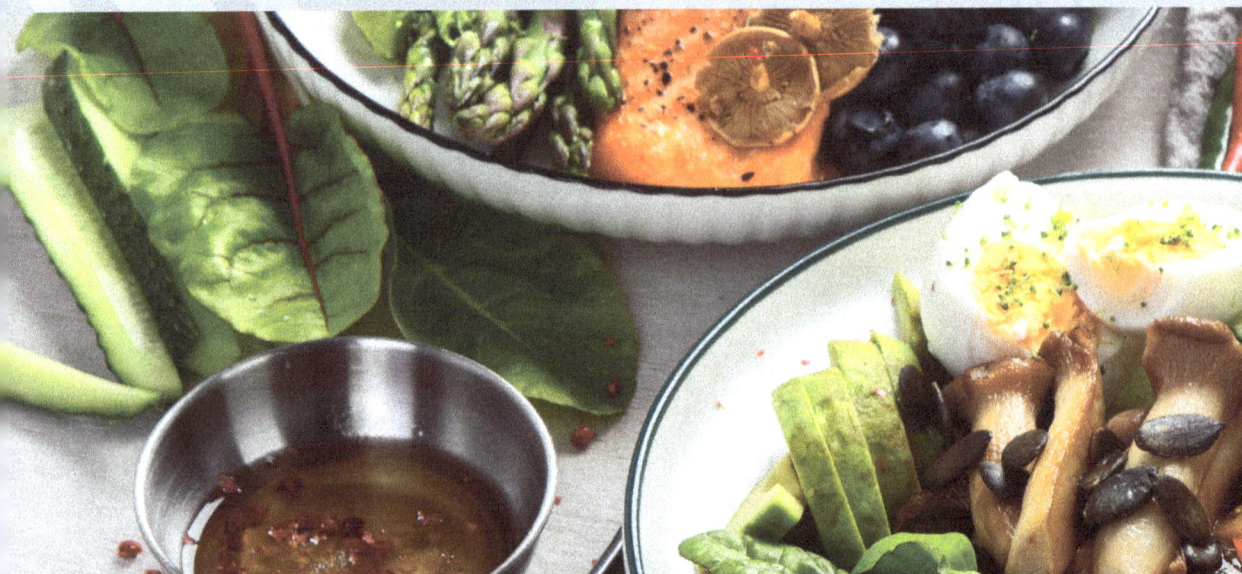

## 5. DRIZZLE WITH A DRESSING OR SAUCE

- Classic Green Goddess (page 154)
- Apple Cider Vinaigrette (page 155)
- Miso-Ginger Dressing (page 154)
- Yogurt-Herb Drizzle (page 155)
- Olive oil + balsamic with sea salt (page 155)
- Coconut aminos + sesame oil (for Asian-style bowls) (page 155)

## 6. FINISH WITH FUN TOPPINGS

- Flax, chia, Zen Basil, hemp seeds
- Toasted pumpkin seeds or sunflower seeds
- Nutritional yeast
- Chopped almonds or walnuts
- Crumbled goat cheese or feta
- Nori strips
- Sauerkraut or kimchi
- Fresh herbs (cilantro, basil, mint, parsley)
- Lemon or lime wedge
- Pickled onions or air-fried onions
- Microgreens

### SUPERWELL PRO TIP

- Want to make this a family night experience? Set up each section buffet-style with signs or cards describing the benefits (e.g., "Greens = fiber & glow"; "Protein = strength & balance").
- **Glow Bowl** – Salmon, quinoa, arugula, rainbow carrots, cucumber, tahini drizzle, hemp seeds
- **Fiesta Bowl** – Ground turkey, brown rice, romaine, tomatoes, corn, avocado-lime sauce
- **Zen Bowl** – Tofu, soba noodles, spinach, shredded cabbage, miso dressing, basil + nori

# SUPERWELL CITRUS-HERB
# *Salmon*

A delicious and zesty take on a dinner staple, this recipe blends omega-rich salmon with citrus and fresh herbs for a flavorful, anti-inflammatory meal that supports heart health, brain function, and glowing skin. With easy air fryer or oven options, it's the kind of dinner that feels fancy without the fuss. Pro tip for our furry friends: Buy salmon with skin on and give the doggies the skin after it has been cooked. SUPERWELL glowing pups . . . salmon skin tastes so good and is great for their coat, skin, and nails!

- 4 wild-caught salmon fillets (6 ounces each)
- Salt to taste
- Black pepper to taste
- 2 tablespoons olive oil or melted ghee
- 1 tablespoon fresh lemon juice
- 1 tablespoon fresh orange juice
- 2 teaspoons manuka honey or maple syrup (optional for a touch of sweetness)
- 2 garlic cloves, minced
- 1 tablespoon fresh dill, chopped (or 1 teaspoon dried dill)
- 1 tablespoon fresh parsley, chopped
- 1 teaspoon smoked paprika
- Lemon and orange slices for garnish

## WHY IT'S SUPERWELL APPROVED

✔ Omega-3 Fatty Acids – Wild-caught salmon is rich in EPA and DHA, essential fats that reduce inflammation, support cognitive health, and contribute to radiant skin and hormone balance.

✔ Citrus Power – Lemon and orange juice deliver vitamin C for immune support and enhanced nutrient absorption.

1. Pat the salmon fillets dry with a paper towel. Season with salt and pepper on both sides.

2. In a small bowl, whisk together olive oil or melted ghee, lemon juice, orange juice, honey or maple syrup (if using), minced garlic, dill, parsley, and smoked paprika.

3. Brush the marinade generously over the salmon fillets. Let them sit for 10–15 minutes to absorb the flavors.

**AIR FRYER INSTRUCTIONS:**

1. Preheat your air fryer to 400°F.

2. Place the salmon fillets in the air fryer basket, skin-side down. Avoid overcrowding.

3. Air fry for 8–10 minutes, depending on the thickness of the fillets, until the salmon is cooked through and flakes easily with a fork.

**OVEN INSTRUCTIONS:**

1. Preheat your oven to 400°F.

2. Place the salmon fillets on a parchment-lined baking sheet, skin-side down.

3. Bake for 12–15 minutes or until the salmon is cooked through and flakes easily.

**SERVE AND ENJOY:**

Garnish with lemon and orange slices for a burst of freshness. Pair with roasted root vegetables, quinoa, or a side of microgreens for a balanced, SUPERWELL meal.

# SUPERWELL SPAGHETTI SQUASH GLOW BOWLS

Comfort food meets functional fuel. These customizable glow bowls deliver pasta-night satisfaction with blood sugar–stabilizing squash, lean protein, and a creamy, gut-friendly sauce. It's everything you love . . . cozy, nourishing, and so delicious!

**YIELD: 2–4 SERVINGS**

1 medium spaghetti squash
1 tablespoon avocado oil or olive oil
Himalayan pink salt to taste
Black pepper to taste
1 cup clean marinara or vodka sauce
1 cup organic low-fat cottage cheese (I love Good Culture)

### *Protein Options*
(Choose at Least One, 1 Cup Total):

Ground turkey
Ground chicken
Ground beef
Ground bison
Cubed grilled chicken
Organic Italian chicken sausage

### *Veggie Add-Ins* (Mix and Match):

Steamed or roasted broccoli
Sautéed spinach or kale
Mushrooms
Zucchini
Shredded carrots
Roasted bell peppers

### *Topping Ideas:*

Fresh basil or parsley
Parmesan cheese or cheese of choice
Crushed red pepper flakes
Nutritional yeast or dairy-free parmesan
Drizzle olive oil or chili oil

### WHY IT'S SUPERWELL APPROVED

- ✔ Spaghetti squash is lower in carbs than pasta, high in fiber and vitamins A and C, and is super satisfying.
- ✔ Cottage cheese is high in protein and creaminess without heavy dairy bloat.
- ✔ Squash shell bake method locks in flavor, cuts down on waste, and feels like comfort food.
- ✔ Protein-focused dish supports satiety, muscle recovery, and blood sugar stability.
- ✔ It's customizable: Clean out your fridge and never get bored with your bowls.

1. Preheat oven to 400°F. Line a baking sheet with parchment.
2. Rinse the squash, cut in half lengthwise, and scoop out the seeds and goo (but leave the good stuff!).
3. Brush the inside with oil and sprinkle with salt and pepper.
4. Place cut-side down, shell up, and roast for 30–45 minutes (depending on the size of the squash), or until fork-tender but still slightly firm (*al dente* texture). **Pro Tip:** Don't over-roast—you want that perfect pastalike *al dente* texture, not mushy. Save the squash shells!
5. Let squash cool for 10–15 minutes. Then use a fork to shred the inside into spaghetti-like strands—the *satisfying autonomous sensory meridian response (ASMR) part!* Scoop shreds into a large mixing bowl. Set shells aside.
6. In a saucepan, gently heat the marinara or vodka sauce with the cottage cheese, stirring until well-blended and creamy. Add salt and pepper to taste.
7. Mix your cooked protein and chopped veggies into the bowl with the shredded spaghetti squash. Pour in the warm sauce and stir everything until fully coated.

## Final Bake
**Optional but Recommended!**

Why This Step Matters:
- Thickens the mixture for better texture
- Locks in flavor
- Prevents wateriness
- Makes it feel like baked pasta

1. Choose your bake vessel.

    *Option 1: Spoon the full mixture back into the squash shells (this makes adorable single-serve portions).*

    *Option 2: Spread into an oven-safe baking dish for a larger, family-style bake.*

2. Top with toppings of choice.
3. Lower the oven temperature to 375°F. Bake for 12–15 minutes, just until warmed through and lightly golden. Optional: Broil for 1–2 minutes for a bubbly finish.
4. Let cool for 5 minutes before serving for the best texture.

## Serving Tip:
- Pack leftovers in meal prep containers for the week—or freeze in shells for ready-to-bake meals on busy days!

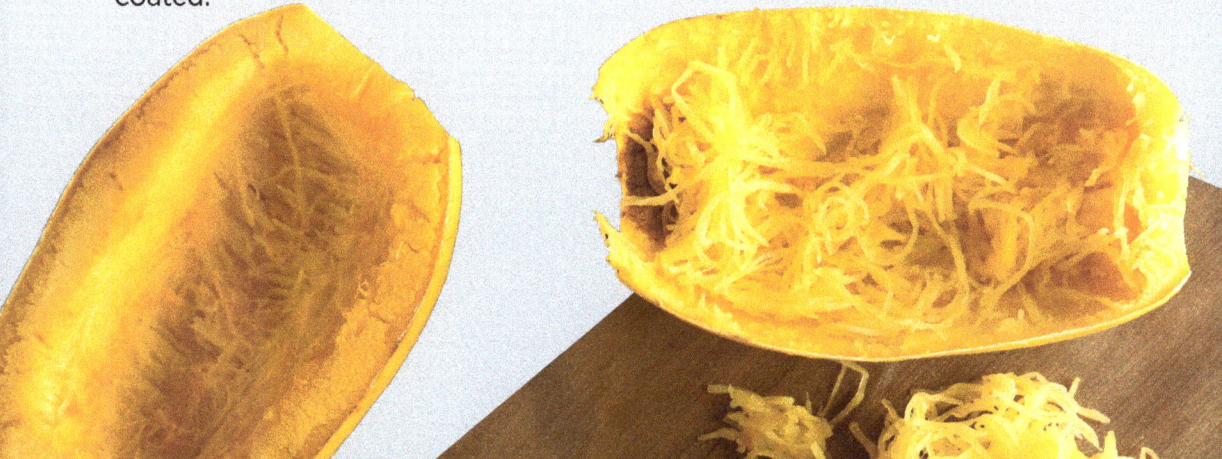

## SUPERWELL ONE-SHEET HARVEST CHICKEN & ROOT VEGGIE DINNER

A family-favorite, one-pan meal that brings together vibrant roasted vegetables, crispy bacon, and herb-crusted chicken for a nourishing dinner that's as easy to make as it is satisfying. The addition of Brussels sprouts elevates the fiber and detox-supporting properties, while the rainbow of root veggies delivers slow-burning carbs and immune-boosting antioxidants. It's the ultimate weeknight dinner—efficient and flavorful!

- 12 bone-in, skin-on chicken thighs
- Himalayan pink salt, to taste
- Cracked black pepper, to taste
- 4 large parsnips, peeled and roll-cut
- 1 large sweet potato, peeled and diced into 1/2-inch cubes
- 1 small butternut squash, peeled and diced into 1/2-inch cubes
- 4 shallots, peeled and cut into thirds
- 2 cups trimmed and halved Brussels sprouts
- 1/4 cup extra virgin olive oil, divided
- 1/2 pound uncured bacon, diced into 1/2-inch pieces
- 3–4 tablespoons finely chopped fresh herbs (rosemary, sage, thyme)

### WHY IT'S SUPERWELL APPROVED

- ✔ **Rainbow Variety:** A medley of root vegetables, shallots, and Brussels sprouts provides fiber, antioxidants, and slow-digesting carbohydrates for hormonal balance and steady energy.
- ✔ **Clean Protein:** Bone-in chicken thighs deliver juicy flavor and lasting satiety, supporting muscle repair and immune health.
- ✔ **Healthy Fats:** Olive oil and bacon add flavor while promoting nutrient absorption and blood sugar stability.
- ✔ **Simple + Strategic:** One pan. No stress. Maximum nourishment. This is SUPERWELL simplicity done right.

1. Preheat oven to 400°F (convection roast, if available). Line two half-sheet pans with parchment paper for easy cleanup.

2. Pat the chicken thighs dry using paper towels (this helps the skin crisp up). Season both sides with salt and pepper. Set aside in a large bowl.

3. In a separate mixing bowl, combine the parsnips, sweet potato, butternut squash, shallots, and Brussels sprouts. Drizzle with 2 tablespoons of the olive oil, and sprinkle with salt and pepper. Toss to coat evenly.

4. Divide the veggie mixture between the two sheet pans, spreading into an even layer. Nestle the seasoned chicken thighs skin-side up over the vegetables.

5. Combine the diced bacon and the chopped herbs in a small bowl. Toss briefly, then distribute the bacon evenly across the chicken and vegetables, making sure pieces aren't clumped together.

6. Drizzle the remaining 2 tablespoons of olive oil over everything on the sheet pans.

7. Roast for 25–35 minutes, or until the chicken reaches an internal temperature of 165°F and the vegetables are fork-tender with golden edges. If desired, broil for the last 2–3 minutes for crispy chicken skin and caramelized veggies.

8. Let rest for 5 minutes before serving. Spoon up generous portions of veggies with each piece of chicken, making sure to include some crispy bacon bits on every plate.

### *Optional Protein Swap:*

Make it your own by swapping chicken thighs for organic drumsticks or bone-in breasts, or serve with wild salmon or grass-fed steak on top of the roasted veggie base.

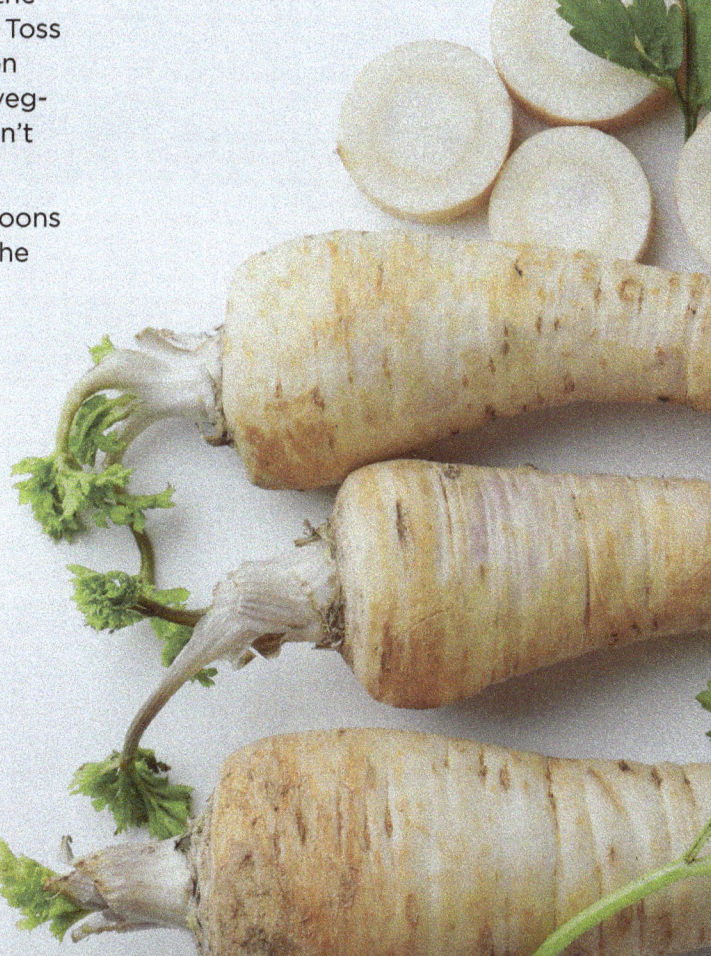

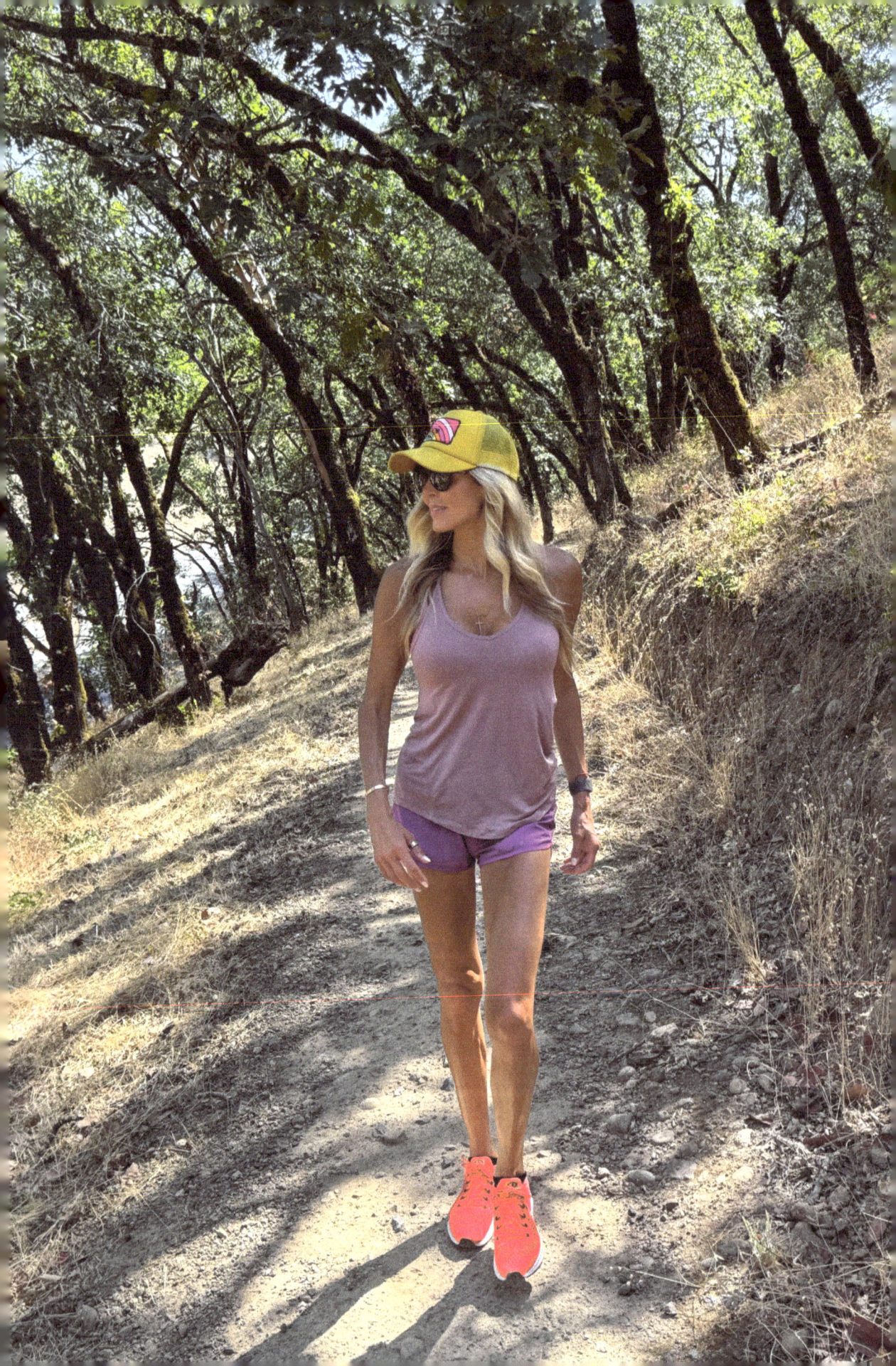

# EVENING WALK MAGIC:
# YOUR SUPERWELL SECRET WEAPON

A walk after dinner may sound simple, but it's one of the most underrated, science-supported practices for long-term metabolic health and one of my non-negotiables. When the sun is setting and the light softens, it's your body's cue to slow down and reset. By syncing your movement with the natural rhythms of the day, you are supporting your circadian clock, the internal 24-hour system that governs everything from hormone production to digestion and sleep cycles.

## GLUCOSE MANAGEMENT STARTS HERE

When you walk after a meal, especially dinner, you are not just burning calories, you are telling your muscles to act like metabolic sponges. After eating, blood glucose levels naturally rise. Rather than letting that sugar linger and spike (which leads to energy crashes, cravings, and even long-term insulin resistance), walking allows your muscles to soak it up efficiently, lowering post-meal glucose and improving insulin sensitivity. This means steadier energy, fewer sugar crashes, and less stress on your pancreas. Just 10–20 minutes of light walking after dinner can significantly blunt the post-meal glucose surge and improve metabolic flexibility.

## A PATH TO BETTER SLEEP

Evening walks also set the tone for more restful sleep. Exposure to natural light, especially the amber glow of sunset, helps your brain produce melatonin at the right time. And when you pair this with gentle movement, you calm your nervous system and regulate cortisol, leading to deeper, more restorative sleep. It's your wind-down ritual in motion.

## MOOD-BOOSTING & STRESS-BUSTING

This isn't just about biology, it's a mental reset too. Moving your body outside after dinner creates a natural buffer between your busy day and the restorative night ahead. Endorphins get released, stress hormones begin to taper, and your mood lifts. It's your time to unplug, breathe deeply, process the day, and prepare to transition both physically and emotionally.

## MY SUPERWELL TIP

I use this walk as a ritualistic reset. Sometimes it's just me and nature. Other times, I walk with Chris or Lilah to connect and reflect. No phone. No tech. Just presence. Add in grounding with bare feet if possible, or simply take off your shoes at the end and pause in stillness.

This isn't just a habit; it's a powerful signal to your body that you are in tune, in control, and creating space to heal, reset, and optimize.

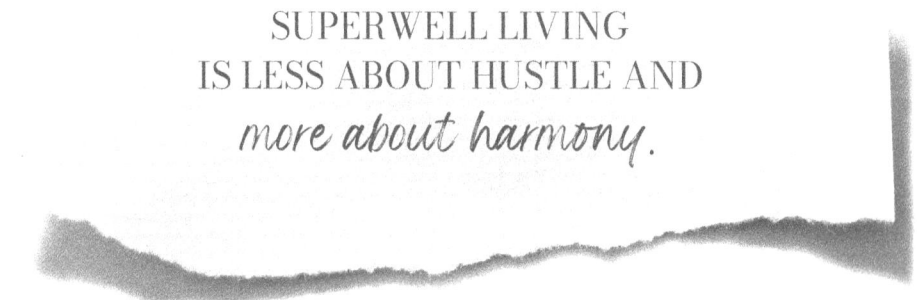

SUPERWELL LIVING IS LESS ABOUT HUSTLE AND *more about harmony.*

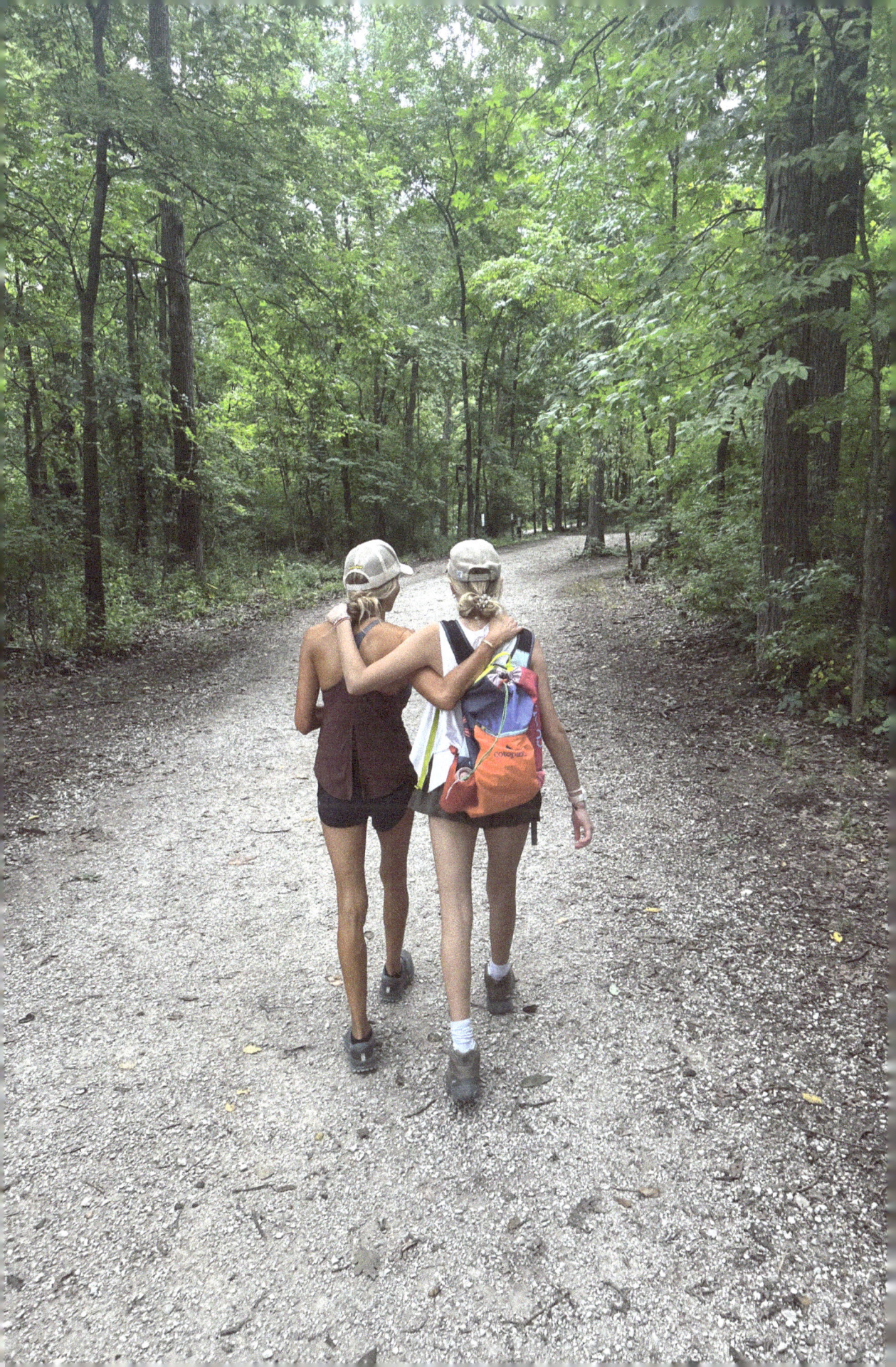

## DIGITAL DIMMING:
# THE SCIENCE & SOUL OF A TECH DETOX

Let's be real; we are tethered to our tech. And while our devices keep us connected and informed, they also hijack the very systems that regulate our energy, emotions, and sleep. That's why I treat my evening tech detox like a non-negotiable wellness boundary, not a restriction. It's one of the most impactful, free tools in my SUPERWELL Living toolkit.

As the sun goes down, our bodies are designed to enter a state of rest and regeneration, but screens tell your brain otherwise. Blue light exposure in the evening has been shown to suppress melatonin production by up to 80%, throwing off your circadian rhythm and delaying deep, restorative sleep. So, that Netflix binge or scroll session before bed? It's not just entertainment; it's a biological disruptor.

## SUPERWELL TIPS FOR A SCIENCE-BACKED DIGITAL WIND DOWN

**Set a Tech Curfew** – I power down all screens by 7:30 P.M. (earlier if I can). This simple habit sends a signal to my brain: It's time to shift from productivity to restoration.

**Blue Light Blockers** – If you absolutely must be on screens after sunset, wear blue-light blocking glasses and activate red light, night shift, or flux settings on your devices. It's not perfect, but it's protective.

**Create a Tech-Free Sanctuary** – Bedrooms are for sleep and connection, not for charging cords, pings, or endless notifications. I charge my phone outside the bedroom and use a Hatch alarm clock, which is a gentle sunrise simulator and sound machine in one. This ensures my sleep space is sacred.

**Dim to Wind Down** – Lower your home lighting in the evening to mimic dusk. Swap overheads for red lights, amber-toned lamps, or Himalayan salt lights to support natural melatonin release.

**Swap Scroll for Stillness** – Replace screen time with rituals that bring your nervous system into balance by reading a real book, meditating, doing breathwork, journaling, stretching, or even just sitting in silence with a calming herbal tea.

## WHY IT MATTERS: THE DEEP BENEFITS OF EVENING TECH BOUNDARIES

**Melatonin Mastery** – Melatonin is your body's internal lullaby, helping you fall asleep faster and stay asleep longer. Reducing screen time allows natural melatonin production to ramp up in the evening, making sleep easier and more effective.

**Mental Clarity & Cognitive Reset** – Endless inputs from screens lead to "mental noise" and emotional dysregulation. Tech detoxing in the evening allows your mind to exhale, process, and reset, supporting memory consolidation and improved cognition overnight.

**CNS Regulation** – The constant stimulation of technology keeps your sympathetic nervous system (fight-or-flight) humming. By unplugging, you activate the parasympathetic (rest-and-digest), allowing your body to calm cortisol, lower heart rate, and prepare for healing.

**Mood & Hormonal Balance** – High screen use at night has been linked to increased stress, disrupted mood, and even elevated nighttime cortisol. By reducing tech exposure, you are supporting not just sleep, but the delicate hormonal harmony that governs everything from metabolism to emotional stability.

**Presence, Not Pressure** – We weren't built to be "on" 24/7. Stepping away from digital stimulation in the evening invites presence, reflection, and real connection both to yourself and to those around you.

# EVENING RITUAL

Create a sanctuary of calm in the evening by indulging in a soothing cup of herbal tea and dimming the lights in your bedroom. This ritual is grounded in science and deeply beneficial for preparing your body for restful sleep. Herbal teas, particularly those containing chamomile, lavender, or valerian root, have been shown to reduce cortisol levels, the stress hormone that can hinder relaxation. Lower cortisol levels promote a state of calm, essential for transitioning from the demands of the day to a restful night. Dimming the lights further enhances this effect by minimizing exposure to artificial light, which can suppress melatonin production. Melatonin is a crucial hormone for regulating your sleep-wake cycle. Together, these practices create a tranquil environment that facilitates the body's natural ability to wind down and achieve restorative sleep. Embrace this calming ritual to end your day on a peaceful note and set yourself up for a rejuvenating night.

## RELAXATION

Herbal tea and dimmed lights create a calming atmosphere, helping to lower cortisol levels. The soothing effects of herbal tea, combined with the gentle ambiance of reduced lighting, foster relaxation and ease stress, making it easier to unwind and prepare for a restful night's sleep.

## SLEEP PREPARATION

A soothing evening ritual signals to your body that it's time to wind down and prepare for sleep. Engaging in calming activities, like sipping herbal tea and dimming the lights, helps establish a routine that cues your body to transition from daytime alertness to nighttime relaxation, promoting a smoother and more restful sleep.

## MIND-BODY CONNECTION

Engaging in a relaxing routine strengthens the mind–body connection, promoting overall wellbeing. By consistently practicing calming activities, you create a harmonious balance between mental and physical states, which enhances relaxation, reduces stress, and supports a healthier, more balanced lifestyle.

## STRESS RELIEF

Herbal teas like chamomile, lavender, and valerian have natural calming properties that help reduce stress. Chamomile promotes relaxation and sleep; lavender has been shown to lower anxiety and enhance calmness; valerian root is a powerful herbal sedative often used to ease tension and improve sleep quality. Sipping these teas in the evening can be a gentle, effective way to unwind and support nervous system balance.

## ENHANCED SLEEP QUALITY

Establishing a consistent evening ritual improves sleep quality and duration. By following a regular, calming routine before bed, you signal to your body that it's time to wind down, which helps regulate your internal clock and prepares you for more restful, uninterrupted sleep. This consistency fosters better sleep habits and can enhance overall sleep satisfaction.

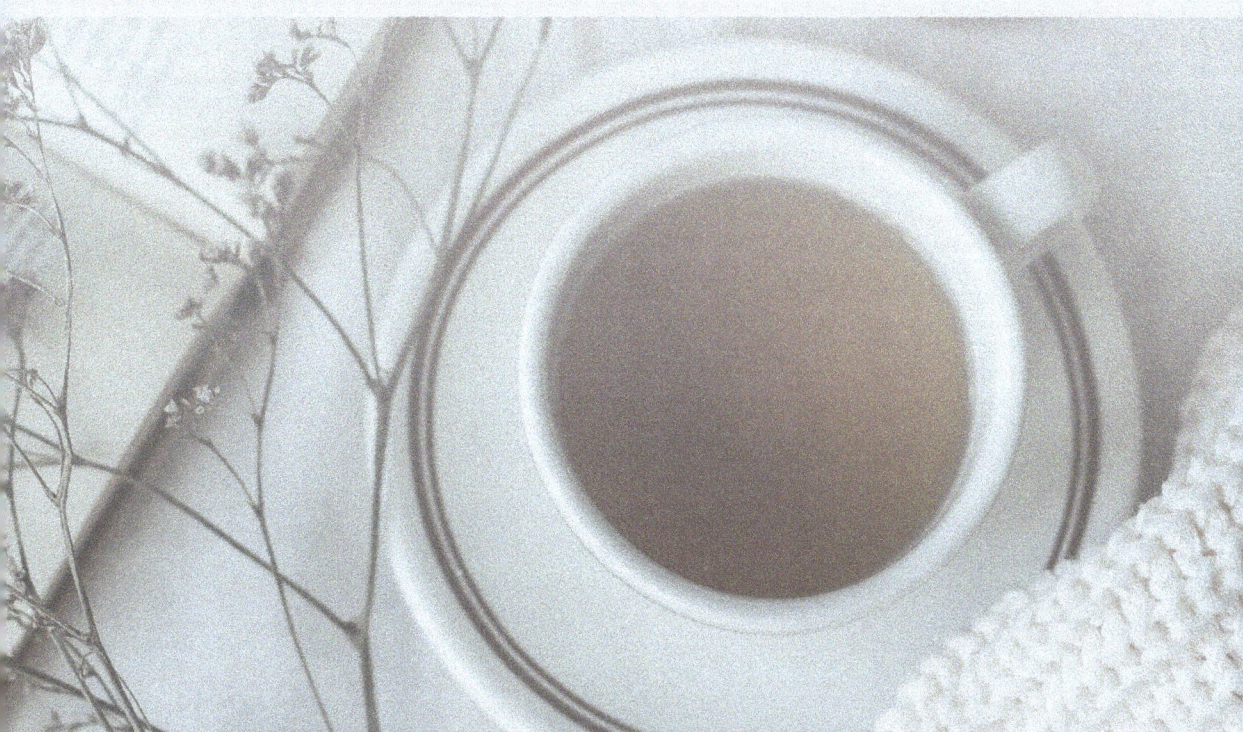

SUPERWELL

# ZEN SLEEP TOOL KIT

**ACUPRESSURE "BED OF NAILS" MAT + PILLOW**

This ancient-inspired tool delivers thousands of tiny pressure points to your back, neck, or feet, activating endorphins and helping to calm an overactive nervous system. By stimulating acupressure meridians, it promotes circulation, reduces cortisol, and releases muscular tension—making it a powerful way to unwind and ground before sleep. Just 10–20 minutes on your "bed of nails" can help melt away the day and ease you into parasympathetic calm.

**WEIGHTED, HEATED, LAVENDER-INFUSED NECK WRAP**

The gentle pressure mimics deep touch stimulation, activating the parasympathetic nervous system. Combined with heat and lavender, it melts muscle tension, lowers cortisol, and signals your body it's time to wind down.

**VAGUS NERVE OIL**

A calming essential oil blend (lavender, chamomile, or neroli) massaged into the neck or behind the ears supports vagal tone. This activates the body's relaxation response, helping reduce anxiety and prepare the mind for rest.

**AROMATHERAPY DIFFUSER WITH ESSENTIAL OILS**

Diffusing grounding scents like sandalwood, vetiver, frankincense, or cedarwood helps lower heart rate, support gamma-aminobutyric acid (GABA) production, and ease the body into deep-wave sleep—ideal for calming the amygdala and balancing cortisol levels.

**RED LIGHT THERAPY BOOK CLIP OR WARM AMBIENT LIGHTING**

Red-spectrum light (600–700 nm) preserves melatonin levels, unlike harsh white or blue light. It's perfect for reading, journaling, or stretching before bed while maintaining circadian alignment.

## SILK SLEEP MASK

Total darkness improves melatonin secretion and sleep cycle regulation. Silk also helps retain skin hydration and reduces irritation around the delicate eye area.

## MOUTH TAPE

Nasal breathing during sleep enhances oxygen uptake, reduces inflammation, supports nitric oxide production, and minimizes disruptions from snoring. It's a simple but game-changing biohack.

## LIGHT CANDLES (BEESWAX OR COCONUT WAX)

Low, warm flickering light signals the brain to power down. Scented with natural oils, it helps set a sacred, calming space to prepare your nervous system for deep rest.

## BLUE LIGHT–BLOCKING GLASSES

Wearing blue light blockers after sunset preserves your melatonin rhythm and minimizes the artificial light exposure that can delay sleep onset and disrupt deep sleep phases.

## PRAYER BEADS

A tactile tool for spiritual grounding or meditation. Whether you're practicing gratitude or reciting mantras, using prayer beads slows breathing, activates alpha brain waves, and soothes bedtime anxiety.

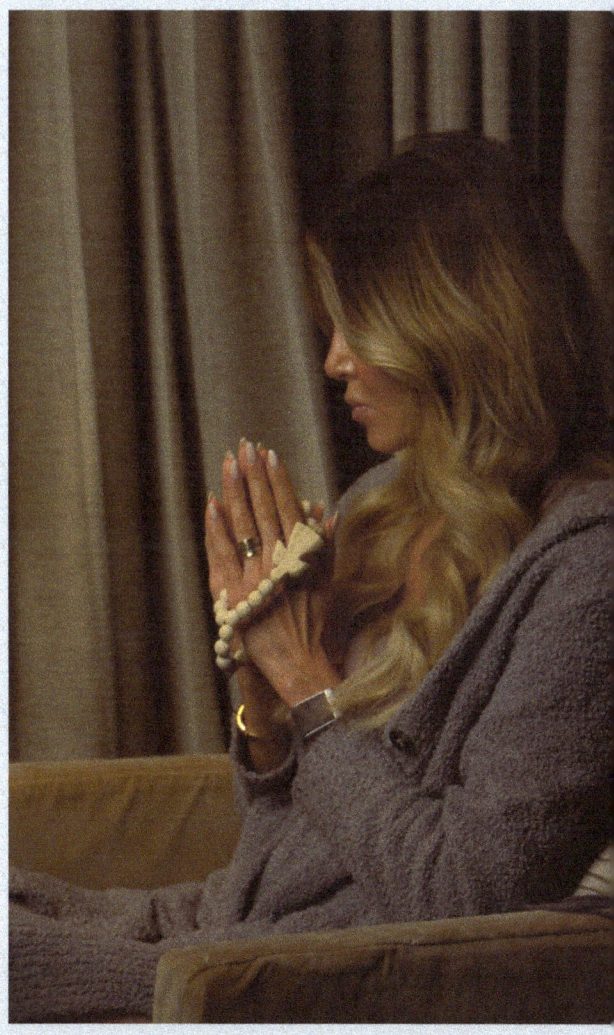

### RED LIGHT BULBS AT BEDSIDE

Switch your nightstand lamp bulbs to red or amber-spectrum bulbs. These support sleep hormone production while providing just enough light to wind down without shocking your nervous system.

### WEIGHTED BLANKET WITH CRYSTAL-INFUSED FILL OR FAR-INFRARED LINING

Upgrade your weighted blanket with natural tourmaline or far-infrared (FIR) materials to balance electromagnetic stress, stimulate serotonin, and promote deeper, restorative sleep through full-body grounding.

### BINAURAL BEATS OR SOLFEGGIO FREQUENCIES

Listening to tracks like 432 hertz or delta wave (0.5–4 Hz) binaural beats can entrain your brain to sleep-supportive states. These audio tools help ease anxious thoughts and support neuroplasticity while you rest.

### CHILLED EYE PILLOW WITH ACUPRESSURE BEADS

Weighted, cool eye masks reduce facial puffiness, calm the optic nerve, and gently stimulate vagus nerve endings to encourage a meditative, sleepy state. They're especially effective post-screen time.

### EARTHING SHEET OR SLEEP MAT

Grounding through conductive bedding connects you to the earth's electrons, reducing nighttime cortisol, inflammation, and electromagnetic field (EMF) exposure. Many report deeper, uninterrupted sleep when consistently used.

### INFRARED HEATING PAD AT FEET OR LOWER BACK

This targeted FIR heat mimics sauna benefits, improving peripheral circulation, reducing muscle tension, and supporting lymphatic flow. It's especially soothing if you've had a high-stress day or physical strain.

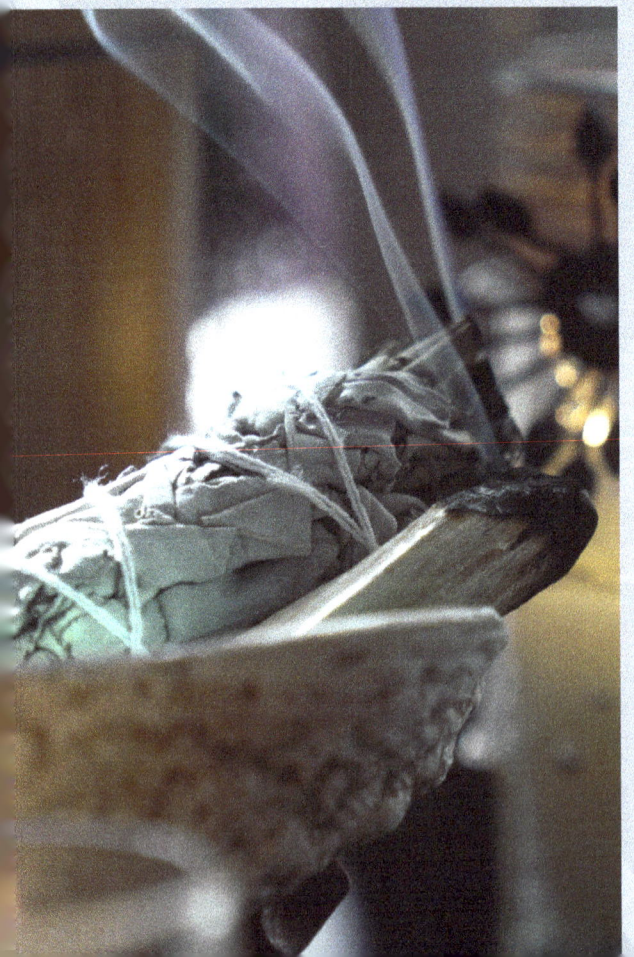

## ADAPTOGENIC HERBAL SLEEP ELIXIRS (SIP RITUAL)

Herbs and supplements like reishi, ashwagandha, passionflower, or magnesium glycinate support adrenal recovery and GABA production. A warm, cozy cup 30–60 minutes before bed helps guide your body into parasympathetic calm.

## TEMPERATURE-REGULATING WEIGHTED COMFORTER

Maintaining an ideal sleeping temperature (around 65°F) is essential for REM sleep. These breathable, cooling-yet-cozy comforters adapt to your body's natural heat fluctuations throughout the night.

## DIGITAL SUNSET ALARM CLOCK (NOT YOUR PHONE!)

This sunrise/sunset simulator gradually dims to mimic dusk, gently easing you into a natural circadian descent. In the morning, it gradually wakes you with soft light, avoiding cortisol spikes from loud alarms or blue screens.

## SANDALWOOD OR CEDARWOOD ON SOLES OF THE FEET

Reflexology meets aromatherapy. These earthy oils activate calming acupressure points and ground overstimulated energy, especially helpful after tech-heavy days or emotional overload.

## MAGNESIUM-INFUSED FOOT SOAK BEFORE BED

A warm foot soak with magnesium flakes (like magnesium chloride or Epsom salts) delivers transdermal relaxation directly where your body absorbs it best—through the feet. Magnesium plays a key role in over 300 enzymatic processes, including calming the nervous system, easing muscle tension, reducing restless leg syndrome, and promoting deep, uninterrupted sleep. Add calming essential oils like lavender or bergamot and soak for 15–20 minutes to fully shift your body into pre-sleep mode.

## BREATHWORK + MEDITATION

I practice 4-7-8 breathing or meditation on my Spoonk mat—legs up the headboard, castor oil pack on my liver, heated pillow on top. This combo activates my vagus nerve, calms my system, and grounds me for deeper sleep.

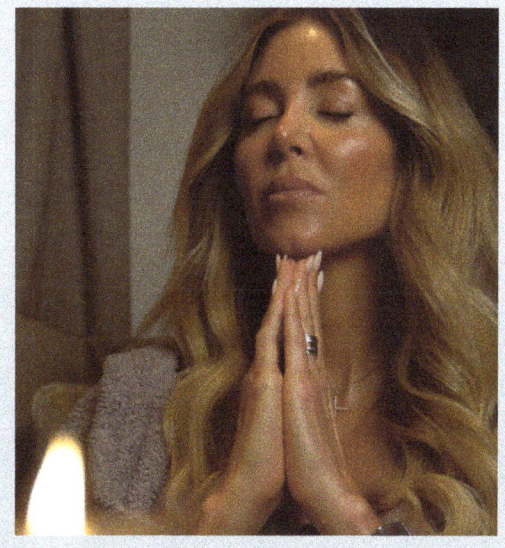

## SUPERWELL TAKEAWAYS

*Master Your Sleep the SUPERWELL Way*

---

### SLEEP HACKS

- Stick to a consistent bedtime.
- Avoid caffeine after noon.
- Skip heavy meals 2 hours before bed.

### SLEEP STACK FOR DEEP REST

- Magnesium: 100–400 milligrams to relax muscles and mind
- Inositol: 1–3 grams to calm your nervous system
- Glycine: 2–3 grams for deeper, restorative sleep
- Better sleep = a better you

### SLEEP LESS, LIVE LESS

- Getting less than 6 hours of sleep increases your risk of heart disease by 48%.
- Sleep deprivation tanks your hormones and wrecks your immune system.
- Sleep is not optional. It's survival.

### SLEEP IS YOUR MOST UNDERRATED FAT LOSS HACK

- Less sleep = more cortisol = more belly fat
- 7–9 hours of quality sleep helps your body burn fat effortlessly.
- Want a lean body? Start with your pillow.

## MAGNESIUM BATH RITUAL:
# A SUPERWELL RESET FOR BODY & MIND

There are few things more healing than a magnesium-infused soak at the end of a long day. This isn't just a bath; it's a thoughtful biochemical recalibration. When I sink into a warm tub with magnesium chloride or Epsom salts, I know I'm giving my body one of the most powerful tools in my recovery arsenal. Magnesium is a key cofactor in over 300 enzymatic reactions, including those involved in muscle repair, energy metabolism, inflammation regulation, and nervous system support. It's no wonder that low magnesium levels are often associated with fatigue, irritability, sleep disruption, and muscle cramps, especially for active women juggling a million responsibilities.

My soak is more than self-care; it's strategy. I habit stack this sacred time with red light, deep breathing, meditation, or even journaling to make it a multi-sensory recharge. Within minutes, the tension melts away as magnesium works transdermally to ease soreness and downshift my nervous system into the parasympathetic rest-and-digest state. This is when true healing begins.

# THE SUPERWELL BENEFITS OF A MAGNESIUM BATH

### MUSCLE RECOVERY

Magnesium supports neuromuscular relaxation by balancing calcium influx in the muscles. This helps prevent cramps, eases soreness, and promotes faster recovery post-workout or post-stress.

### NERVOUS SYSTEM RESET

Transdermal magnesium helps modulate cortisol levels and supports GABA production, the neurotransmitter responsible for calming the brain and promoting sleep.

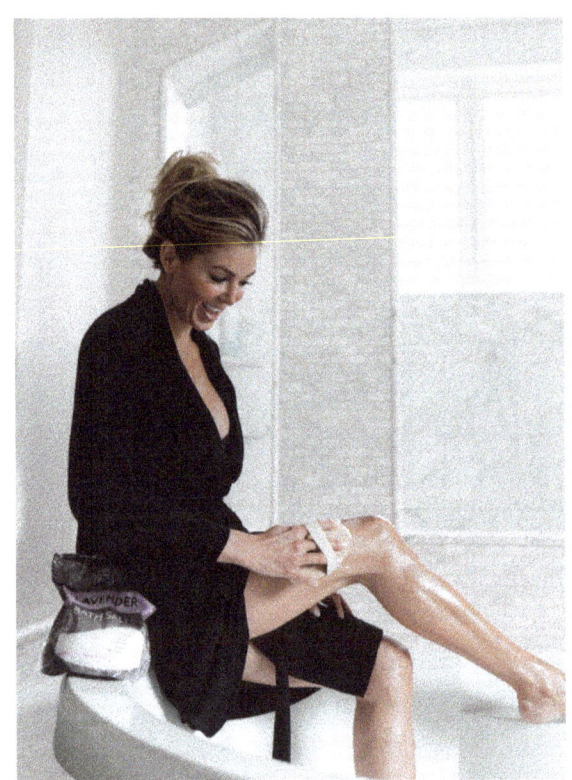

### DETOXIFICATION SUPPORT

The warmth of the bath boosts circulation and induces mild sweating, while magnesium aids the liver in detox pathways. Together, this helps eliminate toxins naturally without overstressing your system.

### SKIN NOURISHMENT

Magnesium has been shown to improve skin hydration, reduce inflammation, and soothe irritated skin. It can be especially beneficial for those with eczema, dry patches, or post-sun exposure irritation.

## DEEPER, RESTORATIVE SLEEP

The magnesium soak not only calms your body but also primes your brain for sleep by enhancing melatonin pathways. I sleep deeper, stay asleep longer, and wake up more refreshed on the nights I soak.

## TIME-SAVING PRO TIP

When I'm short on time, I'll still do a 10-minute magnesium foot soak while I sip a calming herbal tonic and breathe deeply. It may seem simple, but the impact is profound. The secret isn't perfection; it's consistent nourishment and listening to what your body needs most. And sometimes, it just needs a hot bath and silence.

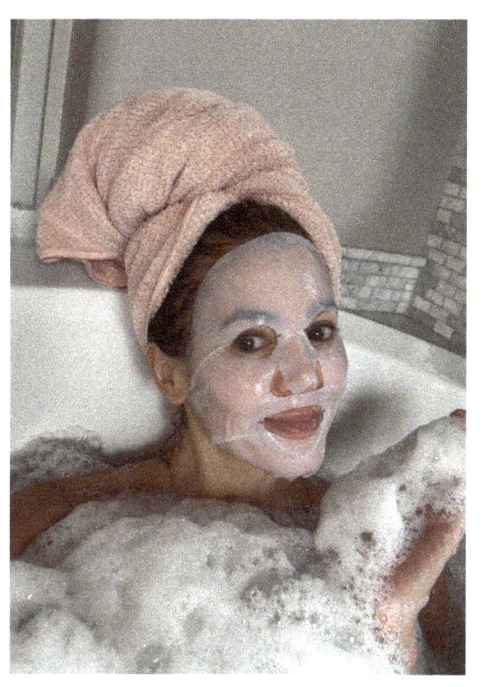

YOUR SUPERWELL GLOW IS YOUR QUIET WAY OF SAYING *I take care of me.*

## PARASYMPATHETIC POWER: MY EVENING MEDITATIVE RESET

Evenings are sacred in my SUPERWELL world—it is a time to shift from doing to being, from output to restoration. One of the most profound ways I have learned to anchor myself into this space is through my meditation practice, a ritual I do twice a day for 20 minutes. I protect this ritual like gold because I have lived both versions of life: in sympathetic overdrive and in parasympathetic ease. And I can tell you, the sweet spot of nervous system regulation lives in the parasympathetic. That's my happy place and where I aim to spend as much time as possible.

Meditation isn't just about relaxation. It's about recalibrating my nervous system, quieting mental chatter, and giving my body a chance to truly repair. This consistent practice doesn't just reduce stress, it reshapes how I respond to life. The science is clear: regular meditation lowers cortisol levels, increases prefrontal cortex activity (hello, decision-making clarity), and enhances the brain's ability to stay calm even during chaos. And here's the secret most people don't realize: doing it twice a day is exponentially more powerful than once. The second session resets the accumulation of stress from the day and primes you for restorative sleep.

I pair this practice with a few of my favorite nighttime recovery tools to create a fully immersive experience. I lie on my "bed of nails"—an acupressure mat that stimulates blood flow, releases natural endorphins, and melts away muscle tension. My legs go up the wall or the headboard, helping drain lymph and reduce swelling. This trifecta of meditation, acupressure, and inversion is a nervous system reset I wish I had discovered sooner, but now it is my gift to you all in creating this blueprint.

## WHY I NEVER SKIP MY EVENING PRACTICE

**Parasympathetic Recalibration** – Meditation activates the vagus nerve, shifting me out of fight-or-flight and into rest-and-digest. This isn't just a buzzword; it's a measurable state that supports digestion, hormone regulation, and cellular repair.

**Enhanced Neuroplasticity** – Studies show that consistent meditation rewires your brain, increasing gray matter in regions associated with memory, empathy, and emotional regulation. These are tools I rely on in every area of life.

**Emotional Resilience** – By creating a buffer between stimulus and reaction, meditation helps me respond to life with grounded calm, rather than reactivity. This shift has transformed not just my wellness, but my relationships.

**Cognitive Clarity & Focus** – TM gives my brain a chance to clear the "mental desktop." I come out of every session more alert, less scattered, and fully re-centered.

**Sleep Onset & Quality** – Meditation before bed has been shown to increase melatonin levels naturally and reduce the time it takes to fall asleep. I drift off more peacefully and stay asleep longer, waking up with energy that feels earned, not forced.

**Pro Tip:** – I often stack this ritual with essential oils (vetiver and sandalwood are my go-to), soft lighting, and a few deep 4-7-8 breaths before I begin. I have turned my bedroom into a CNS reset sanctuary, and it starts with this non-negotiable 20 minutes.

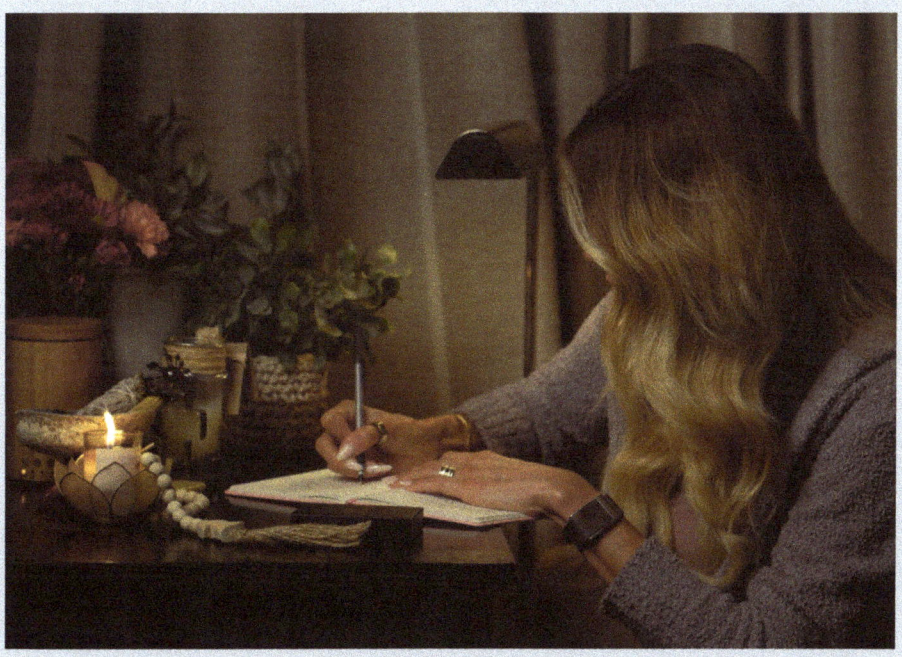

# MY SUPERWELL NIGHTTIME RITUAL

*The Ultimate Nervous System Wind-Down + Skin Rejuvenation Stack*

This routine is more than just relaxation; it's my nightly nervous system reset. It allows my body to fully transition from high-performance mode into deep, healing recovery so I can wake up energized, restored, and glowing from the inside out.

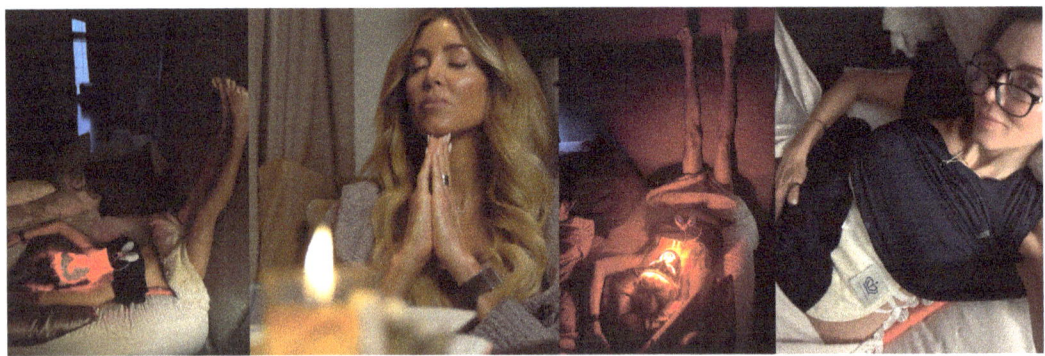

### LED RED LIGHT FACE & NECK MASK

I use this clinically-backed tool to promote collagen production, reduce fine lines, and increase cellular energy (ATP) in the skin. Red and near-infrared wavelengths penetrate deeply to support mitochondrial health, calm inflammation, and accelerate skin repair, an effortless way to rejuvenate while I unwind.

### 4-7-8 OR BOX BREATHING TECHNIQUE

While the red light works its magic, I pair it with controlled breathwork to guide my body into a parasympathetic state. Breath practices like 4-7-8 slow the heart rate, lower cortisol, and enhance vagal tone, acting like a gear shift that signals my nervous system it's time for deep rest.

## LEGS UP THE WALL (VIPARITA KARANI)

This simple inversion helps drain lymphatic fluid, reduce lower-body inflammation, and calm the adrenal glands. It enhances venous return, improves circulation, and supports hormone balance, all while encouraging the body to shift into restoration mode.

## CASTOR OIL PACK WITH HEATED NECK PILLOW

Castor oil is a time-honored remedy known for its anti-inflammatory and liver-supporting properties. The gentle heat amplifies absorption, promotes detoxification, and soothes the gut-brain connection, making it one of my favorite tools to calm digestion and prep for quality sleep.

## ACUPRESSURE "BED OF NAILS" MAT

Lying on this mat stimulates endorphin release and promotes myofascial relaxation, targeting pressure points along the spine to calm tension and rebalance energy. It mimics the therapeutic benefits of acupuncture, encouraging the body to enter a state of healing and renewal.

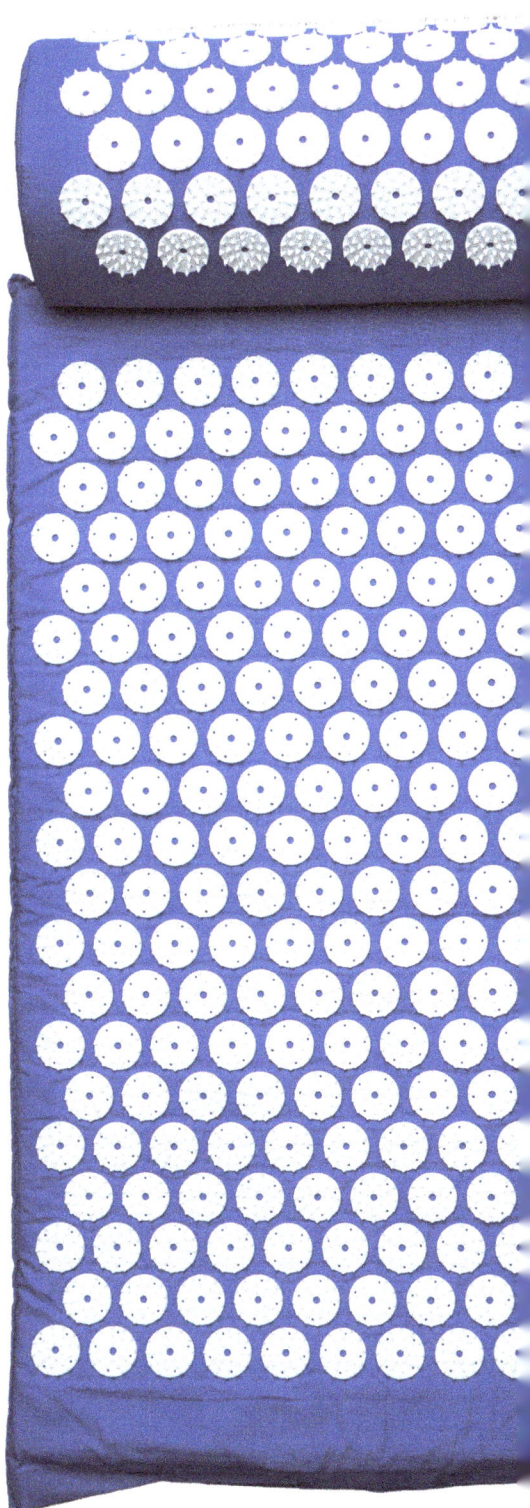

SUPERWELL GLOWING SKIN
P.M. ROUTINE

# RETINOL & ACID SLOUGH-OFF NIGHTS

## FOR ULTIMATE CELL TURNOVER, RENEWAL, & RADIANCE

These exfoliation and renewal nights are just as important as my TLC hydration nights. Think of them as the "workouts" for your skin, encouraging cellular renewal, refining texture, and keeping the skin clear, bright, and firm. I alternate these cell turnover/slough-off nights with my deep hydration routine, ensuring a balanced cycle between exfoliation, renewal, and replenishment. I alternate between these nights depending on what my skin is telling me when I look in the mirror. It's always changing depending on travel, stress, and seasons. This is where we challenge the skin while still keeping it strong and resilient.

## THE POWER OF RETINOL & ACIDS: WHY YOU NEED SLOUGH-OFF NIGHTS

- Speeds up cell turnover, revealing fresher, healthier skin.
- Stimulates collagen and elastin, preventing wrinkles and sagging.
- Unclogs pores and prevents breakouts, which is essential for clear, refined skin.
- Brightens and evens out skin tone, fading hyperpigmentation and sun damage.

# HOW I MAXIMIZE RETIN-A & ACIDS WITHOUT COMPROMISING MY SKIN BARRIER

## STEP 1: CLEANSE & PREP THE SKIN

### *Cleanser:*

May Lindstrom
The Pendulum Potion

- Oil-based and gentle—doesn't strip the skin.
- Removes sunscreen, dirt, and makeup effectively.
- Prepares the skin for treatment without over-drying.

### *How to Use:*

1. Massage 1-2 pumps into dry skin.
2. Take your time to do lymphatic drainage massage—this helps detox the skin.
3. Rinse and pat dry with Clean Skin Club antibacterial towels.

*Pro Tip:*
If your skin is sensitive to retinol, use a gentle, non-exfoliating cleanser on these nights.

## STEP 2: WAIT FOR SKIN TO FULLY DRY

### *Why?*

Applying Retin-A (Tretinoin) on damp skin increases absorption and can lead to irritation. Let your skin dry for at least 10-15 minutes before applying actives.

### *What to Do While Waiting?*

- Apply castor oil pack and put legs up the wall.
- Breathwork, meditation, or journaling.
- Hydration break—sip on herbal tea or water.

## STEP 3: APPLY RETIN-A (TRETINOIN) 0.05%

### Why?

Tretinoin (Retin-A) is the gold standard in dermatology for:

- Reducing fine lines and wrinkles
- Clearing acne and preventing breakouts
- Boosting collagen production
- Improving skin texture and tone

### How to Use

1. Take a pea-sized amount (yes, that's all you need for your face and neck).
2. Dot it on the forehead, cheeks, chin, and neck.
3. Gently spread it across the skin—do not rub in aggressively.

### Alternative for Those Who Can't Tolerate Retin-A

- Retinol (weaker, but still effective), like SkinCeuticals Retinol 0.3% or 0.5%
- Bakuchiol (natural alternative), like Omorovicza Miracle Facial Oil
- Gentle exfoliating acids (see below)

### Pro Tip:

**The Sandwich Method (For Beginners)**

If you are new to tretinoin or have sensitive skin, buffer it with a barrier cream:

1. Apply a light moisturizer first (like La Roche-Posay Cicaplast Baume B5 or Vanicream).
2. Then, apply your tretinoin.
3. Follow up with another moisturizer to lock it in.

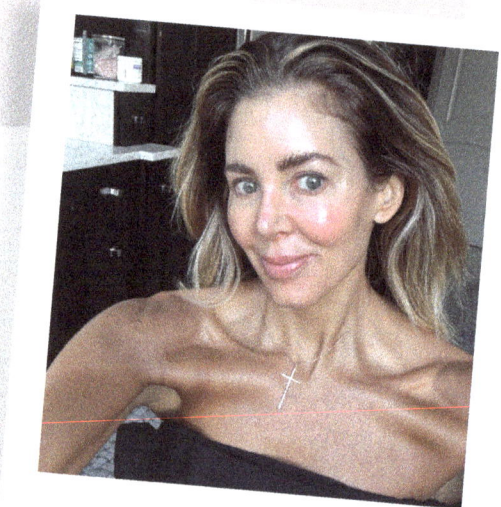

## STEP 4: NECK & CHEST CARE

*RFA Koji Clear Pads*

Swipe across neck and chest (brightening and tone-evening).

*RFA Youthful Neck Cream*

Firms and tightens neck and décolleté.

*Why Treat Your Neck & Chest?*

The skin here is thinner and ages faster, so it needs the same care as your face!

## STEP 5: LIP CARE & FINAL TOUCHES

*Lips:*

Dr. Dennis Gross Derm Infusion Plump & Repair Lip Treatment
Hydrates, plumps, and repairs overnight.

*Final Step:*

If needed, apply a thin layer of La Roche-Posay Cicaplast Baume B5 to lock in moisture and reduce irritation from tretinoin.

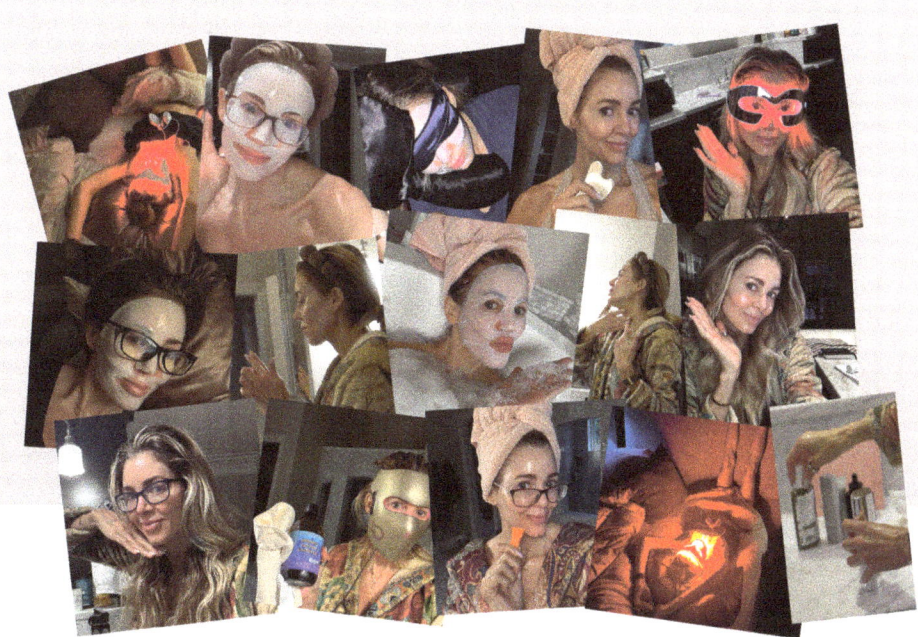

## ALTERNATE WITH AN EXFOLIATING ACID NIGHT (INSTEAD OF TRETINOIN)

If your skin can't tolerate retinoids or you want to switch things up, use an exfoliating acid night instead.

### Best Acids for Exfoliation & Glow

- Mandelic acid (gentle, great for sensitive skin), like Allies of Skin Mandelic Pigmentation Corrector
- Lactic acid (hydrating, great for dull skin), like Sunday Riley Good Genes
- Glycolic acid (stronger, resurfaces skin), like Dr. Dennis Gross Alpha Beta Peel Pads
- Salicylic acid (for acne-prone skin), like Paula's Choice 2% BHA Liquid Exfoliant

### How to Use Acid Nights

- Apply exfoliating serum or pad to dry skin after cleansing.
- Let absorb for 2–3 minutes before layering moisturizer.
- Do *not* use Retin-A and exfoliating acids on the same night.

## HYDRATION & BARRIER SUPPORT

After Retin-A or an acid night, your skin needs extra hydration and barrier repair.

### Hydrating Mist

Eminence Stone Crop Hydrating Mist

- Locks in moisture and preps skin for next steps.
- Use 2–3 spritzes between each step.

### Moisturizer

RFA Hydra Lipid Moisturizer or Epionce Intensive Nourishing Night Cream

- Strengthens skin barrier and prevents irritation.
- Hydrates without clogging pores.

### Pro Tip:

If your skin feels extra dry, add a drop of face oil (like Le Prunier Plum Oil) on top of your moisturizer.

## HOW TO GET USED TO TRETINOIN—THE ULTIMATE TOLERANCE PLAN

If you are new to tretinoin, here is how to build tolerance without irritation:

- **Start Slow:** Apply only 2 times per week at first (e.g., Mondays and Thursdays).
- **Use a Buffer:** Apply a moisturizer first before tretinoin for the first 2–4 weeks.
- **Increase Gradually:** After a month, move to 3x per week, then 4x, and eventually every other night.
- ***Always* Moisturize:** Hydrated skin tolerates retinol better.
- **Never Skip SPF:** Retin-A makes skin sun-sensitive. Always use SPF 50+ during the day.

## *Final Thoughts:*
## *Why Slough-Off Nights Are Non-Negotiable*

You will wake up with smoother, brighter, and firmer skin.

It prevents clogged pores, dullness, and uneven texture.

Over time, these nights will be the secret to long-term skin renewal and glow.

Balance is key—challenge your skin, but don't overdo it.

Listen to your skin and adjust accordingly.

Pair this with your hydration nights for the ultimate SUPERWELL glow!

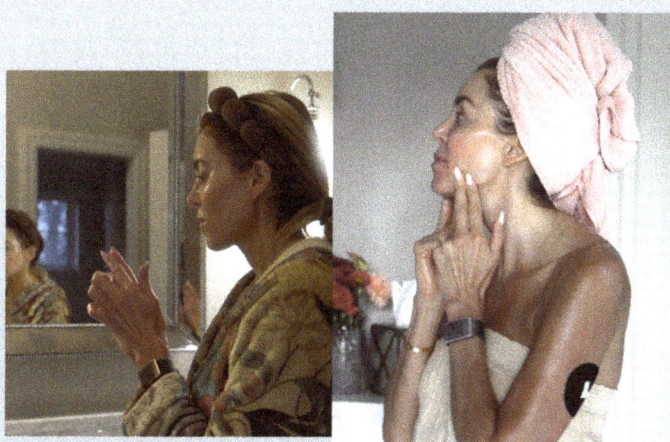
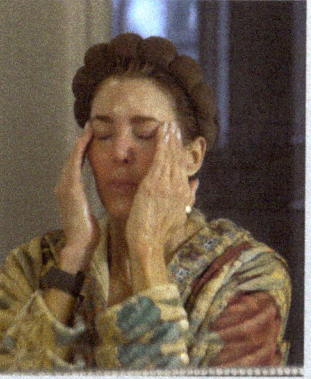

# SMART SUPPLEMENTATION + NOURISHMENT

Optimize your nightly recovery ritual with a strategic blend of supplementation and relaxation practices that align with your body's natural rhythm. I'm a firm believer in getting the bulk of your vitamins, minerals, and phytonutrients from nutrient-dense, whole foods because the synergy of real food is something no capsule can replicate. Also, understand that today's modern world and depleted soil often leave nutritional gaps even in the cleanest diets.

That is where intentional, high-quality supplements come in, not as a crutch, but as a smart enhancement. I keep my blueprint supplement routine minimal and meaningful, carefully selecting only what supports my unique bio-individual needs based on lab work, energy levels, sleep quality, and nervous system resilience.

In the evenings, I turn to magnesium glycinate, a key mineral that supports over 300 enzymatic processes in the body, including muscle recovery, neurotransmitter balance, and the production of GABA, the calming neurotransmitter that helps initiate sleep. It's foundational for a calm mind and body. I also take ashwagandha, a time-tested adaptogen that helps regulate cortisol, rebalance stress hormones, and support my body's ability to wind down naturally.

For beauty from within, I have found great value in collagen-rich blends and clean skin-hair-nail supplements that support cellular repair while I sleep, when our body is naturally in restoration mode. But remember, the true magic happens when these are paired with real nourishment: leafy greens, omega-rich seeds, wild salmon, bone broth, and vibrant plants from nature's apothecary.

To amplify the effects, I apply calming essential oils like lavender, vetiver, or chamomile behind the ears and on the back of my neck to stimulate the vagus nerve, creating a cascade of relaxation signals throughout the body. This, along with my nightly rituals, forms my blueprint for a holistic sleep sanctuary in caring for my mind, body, and spirit with reverence.

Less is more when it comes to supplements. Know your body. Trust your gut. And always start with real food. Supplements should *support* your wellness, not *define* it.

## NUTRITIONAL BOOST

Supplements provide essential nutrients that support overall health and wellbeing. By filling nutritional gaps and enhancing your diet, they help maintain optimal bodily functions, boost energy levels, and promote a balanced and healthy lifestyle.

## RELAXATION

Magnesium supplements help relax muscles and nerves, promoting better sleep. By supporting muscle relaxation and calming the nervous system, magnesium can make it easier to unwind and fall asleep, contributing to more restful and restorative nights.

## HAIR HEALTH

Certain supplements support healthy hair growth and reduce shedding. Nutrients such as biotin, zinc, and vitamins A and D play crucial roles in strengthening hair follicles, promoting growth, and minimizing hair loss, helping you maintain a fuller, healthier mane.

## NERVE FUNCTION

Applying oil to the vagus nerve area can promote relaxation and reduce tension. The gentle massage and soothing properties of the oil help stimulate the vagus nerve, which plays a key role in calming the nervous system and alleviating stress, leading to a deeper sense of relaxation and tranquility.

## OVERALL WELLNESS

Incorporating supplements into your routine ensures you are nourishing your body from the inside out. By providing essential nutrients that may be missing from your diet, supplements help support overall health, enhance bodily functions, and contribute to a well-rounded approach to wellness.

# SUPERWELL
## Slumber Sipper

*Calm Your Body, Clear Your Mind, Sleep Like You Mean It*

This isn't just a bedtime drink—it's an intentional wind-down ritual designed to support your nervous system, stabilize hormones, and prime your body for deep, restorative rest. Packed with multi-sourced magnesium, naturally occurring melatonin, and calming adaptogens, this elixir is your nighttime ally for metabolic repair, cognitive reset, and that radiant morning glow. Cherry juice is a natural source of melatonin and is antioxidant-rich; lemon juice adds liver and digestion support; and pink Himalayan salt adds electrolyte replenishment and cellular hydration.

My favorite? Magnesi-Om Berry Flavor by Moon Juice—a blend of three highly absorbable types of magnesium + L-theanine to smooth stress, relax tight muscles, and help your body transition into true parasympathetic recovery. This ritual isn't just about sleep; it's about restoring your whole system and setting the stage for tomorrow's glow. SUPERWELL sleep starts here!

**YIELD: 1 SERVING**

- 1 teaspoon Moon Juice Magnesi-Om Berry Flavor (or your favorite clean magnesium powder blend)
- 2 ounces tart cherry juice
- Juice of 1 lemon
- 1 dropper full of liquid ashwagandha or tulsi extract (optional for extra cortisol regulation and calm)
- Pinch of pink Himalayan salt
- 10 ounces sparkling mineral water or warm still water (depending on your mood)
- Fresh mint sprig, black cherries, or dried edible rose petals for a SUPERWELL signature glow (optional garnish)

SUPERWELL RECIPES

1. In a glass or cozy mug, stir together Magnesi-Om, tart cherry juice, lemon juice, and adaptogens (if using).
2. Add a pinch of pink salt and top with your choice of warm still water or sparkling mineral water.
3. Gently stir and garnish with a sprig of mint, black cherries, or rose petals (if using).
4. Sip slowly, breathe deeply, and let this become your new nightly rhythm for healing and harmony.

## WHY IT'S SUPERWELL APPROVED

✔ Multi-magnesium complex supports nervous system regulation, muscle repair, and deep sleep cycles.

✔ Tart cherry juice naturally boosts melatonin and helps reduce inflammation.

✔ Lemon + pink salt support detox, mineral balance, and overnight hydration.

✔ Adaptogens like tulsi or ashwagandha help lower cortisol and calm the mind.

## SUPERWELL ADULT HOT CHOCOLATE

Warm up with this decadent and protein-packed treat! This rich and chocolatey drink makes it easy to enjoy a protein boost while satisfying your cravings for a cozy, sweet treat on a cold day.

1 cup unsweetened vanilla almond milk or milk of choice

1/2 cup (1 scoop) Paleo Valley Chocolate Bone Broth Protein

1 tablespoon maple syrup (optional for added sweetness)

Dash of cinnamon (for garnish)

1. Heat the almond milk in a small saucepan over medium heat until warm but not boiling.
2. Whisk in the chocolate bone broth protein until smooth and creamy.
3. Stir in maple syrup for extra sweetness, if using.
4. Pour into a mug and sprinkle with a dash of cinnamon for a cozy finish.

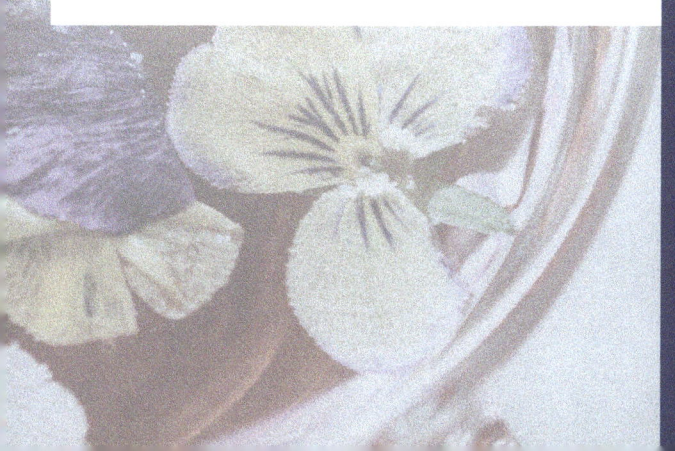

# LITERARY ESCAPE

Immerse yourself in a captivating book before bed to enhance your nightly routine and improve sleep quality. Engaging with printed material rather than digital screens reduces exposure to blue light, which is known to suppress melatonin production and interfere with your body's natural sleep-wake cycle. This shift away from screens fosters a more tranquil mental state, preparing your mind for restful sleep.

Enhance this ritual by using a red light therapy clip book light. Red light has been scientifically shown to minimize disruption to circadian rhythms and support the natural sleep process, making it an ideal companion for nighttime reading. As you dive into different worlds and perspectives, you not only escape the stresses of the day but also benefit from a calming, sleep-promoting environment.

By integrating these practices into your evening routine, you create a serene and restorative atmosphere that encourages deep, rejuvenating sleep, setting the stage for a refreshed start to the next day.

## MENTAL HEALTH

Reading before bed is a powerful tool for mental regulation. Studies show that even 6 minutes of reading can reduce stress levels by up to 68%, calming the nervous system and decreasing cortisol levels. Engaging with a book allows the mind to disengage from external stimuli and looping thoughts, promoting emotional decompression and inner stillness as you transition into sleep.

## IMAGINATION

Literature activates neural networks tied to creativity, empathy, and visualization. As your brain constructs scenes, interprets characters, and fills in narrative gaps, it exercises the prefrontal cortex and default mode network, which are key areas associated with creative thinking and emotional processing. This kind of imaginative stimulation fosters neuroplasticity and supports more dynamic problem solving in daily life.

## COGNITIVE FUNCTION

Reading regularly is linked to long-term cognitive resilience and brain longevity. The mental effort required to follow plotlines, recall character development, and integrate themes strengthens working memory and neural connections. Over time, this "mental resistance training" may lower the risk of age-related cognitive decline and enhance executive functioning across all areas of life.

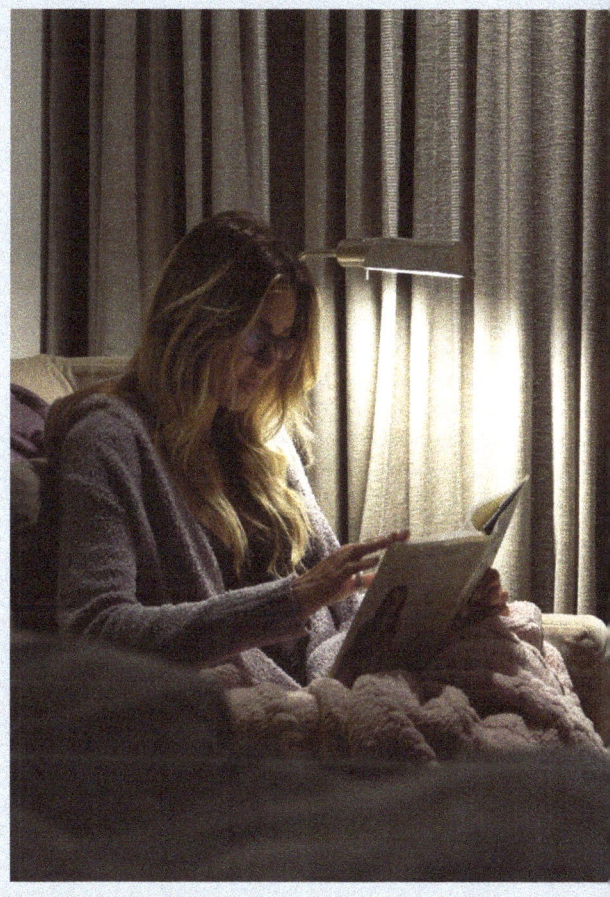

## STRESS REDUCTION

Immersing yourself in a well-written story offers a form of meditative escapism that allows the body to exit fight-or-flight mode. Reading slows the heart rate, eases muscle tension, and quiets mental chatter, which are essential for rebalancing the nervous system. This nightly retreat helps reset the body's stress response and signals safety, which is crucial for hormonal regulation and recovery.

## IMPROVED SLEEP

As part of your evening routine, reading becomes a circadian cue that tells your brain it's time to wind down, unlike screen exposure, which disrupts melatonin production and delays sleep onset. Reading a physical book under soft lighting (or even better, red light) supports healthy sleep architecture. This habit promotes a smoother transition into deep, restorative sleep and enhances overnight memory consolidation.

# SUPERWELL READS

**GOOD ENERGY:**
*The Surprising Connection Between Metabolism and Limitless Health*
By Dr. Casey Means

**THE LIGHT WORK:**
*Reclaim Your Feminine Power, Live Your Cosmic Truth, and Illuminate the World*
By Jessica Zweig

**THE NEW MENOPAUSE:**
*Navigating Your Path Through Hormonal Change with Purpose, Power, and Facts*
By Mary Claire Haver

**PRESENT OVER PERFECT:**
*Leaving Behind Frantic for a Simpler, More Soulful Way of Living*
By Shauna Niequist

**100 WAYS TO CHANGE YOUR LIFE:**
*The Science of Leveling Up Health, Happiness, Relationships & Success*
By Liz Moody

**THE GIFTS OF IMPERFECTION:**
*Let Go of Who You Think You're Supposed to Be and Embrace Who You Are*
By Brené Brown

**GUT FEELINGS:**
*Healing the Shame-Fueled Relationship Between What You Eat and How You Feel*
By Dr. Will Cole

**THE 5 TYPES OF WEALTH:**
*A Transformative Guide to Design Your Dream Life*
By Sahil Bloom

**THINK LIKE A MONK:**
*Train Your Mind for Peace and Purpose Every Day*
By Jay Shetty

**OUTLIVE:**
*The Science and Art of Longevity*
By Peter Attia, MD

**FOREVER STRONG:**
*A New, Science-Based Strategy for Aging Well*
By Dr. Gabrielle Lyon

**ATOMIC HABITS:**
*An Easy and Proven Way to Build Good Habits & Break Bad Ones*
By James Clear

# LIGHTS OUT: YOUR EVENING BLUEPRINT FOR SUPERWELL SLEEP

The true foundation of SUPERWELL Living starts not in the morning, but the night before. A well-rested body is a high-performing body, and deep, restorative sleep is non-negotiable for optimal energy, hormone regulation, cognitive performance, and emotional resilience. That's why I treat sleep like the sacred ceremony it is, with intention and alignment every single night.

I aim to wind down around 9 P.M., in rhythm with my body's natural circadian biology. This is when melatonin naturally begins to rise; it's your internal signal that it's time to recover, restore, and renew. My bedroom temperature is always set between 66–67°F, because lowering your core body temperature helps stimulate sleep onset and enhances REM sleep quality. Too warm? You are likely interrupting the deep sleep cycles needed for full cellular repair.

I also avoid eating within 2–3 hours of bedtime. Based on my continuous glucose monitoring and heart rate variability (HRV) data, eating too close to sleep disrupts both insulin sensitivity and overnight heart rate variability. That means less deep sleep, more inflammation, and sluggish recovery the next day. Instead, I close my eating window early (usually by 5:30 or 6 P.M.), allowing my body to enter a deeper parasympathetic state where digestion is done and healing begins.

Sleep isn't just about quantity, it's about quality and intention. Every element of my bedtime routine is a cue to the body: *You are safe, you are supported, you can fully let go.*

When you prioritize your recovery, everything else becomes easier—your workouts, your emotional regulation, your creativity, your joy. And that is what SUPERWELL Living is truly about.

# CONCLUSION: THE JOURNEY TO SUPERWELL—TOGETHER

## This Is Just the Beginning

If there is one thing I want you to take away from this book, it's this: The journey to SUPERWELL is never-ending, and you are never walking it alone.

Each day is a new opportunity and a chance to wake up and decide how you will show up for yourself. Some days, that choice feels effortless. Other days, it feels like an uphill battle. But no matter where you are in your journey, remember this: You are in control. You are the well. You have the power to fill it, nourish it, and sustain it.

### THE POWER OF DAILY CHOICES

I am not a doctor. I do not claim to have all the answers or a magic formula for perfect health. But what I do have is a relentless passion for learning, experimenting, and sharing what works. Every day, I push myself to explore new ways to optimize my health, whether it's biohacking, contrast therapy, meditation, or simply getting back to the basics of movement, nutrition, and rest. I am my own guinea pig, constantly testing, tweaking, and evolving.

And here's what I have learned: Our health is not written in stone. Genetics may load the gun, but our daily choices pull the trigger. This is epigenetics in action, which is the science that proves our lifestyle, habits, and environment influence how our genes express themselves. You and I may have predispositions to disease, but that does not mean we are powerless. Every mindful choice we make—from the foods we eat, to the breath we take, to the way we move, think, and rest—has the power to shape our future.

That's exactly why this book was written not as a one-size-fits-all plan, but as *your* ultimate *blueprint*—a living, breathing framework to help you build sustainable habits that serve your body and your life. One page at a time. One habit at a time.

This is not about achieving perfection. It's about striving, because the beauty of this journey is that there is always room to grow, to improve, and to evolve. That is what keeps life exciting. That is what keeps us striving for more.

## YOU ARE NOT ALONE

Throughout this book, I have shared my story, my struggles, my wins, and the lessons I have learned along the way. But this is not just about me; it's about all of us. We are in this together.

So, consider me your SUPERWELL Living BFF—your cheerleader, your guide, and your accountability partner. Whether you are just starting out or fine-tuning your wellness rhythm, I am here, walking this path right alongside you.

Every time you wake up and choose to drink the water, breathe deeply, step into the sunlight, move your body, fuel it well, rest when needed, and surround yourself with people who lift you up, you are choosing to follow your *blueprint*. You are choosing to strive for SUPERWELL. And I will be right here, continuing to learn, grow, and share with you every step of the way.

**THIS IS JUST THE BEGINNING**

The journey to SUPERWELL does not end with this book; it is a lifestyle, a mindset, a commitment to never settling for just "well" when you can feel truly alive.

So let's keep going, together. Let's continue to learn, to challenge ourselves, to embrace both the science and the art of wellbeing. Let's wake up each day with the mindset that we are the well—striving, always striving, to be SUPERWELL.

Thank you for walking this path with me. Now go out there and live it.

With Warmth & Wellness,
Your SUPERWELL BFF,

*Lauren*

THE SUPERWELL METHOD REMINDS US *wellness is a rhythm, not a race.*

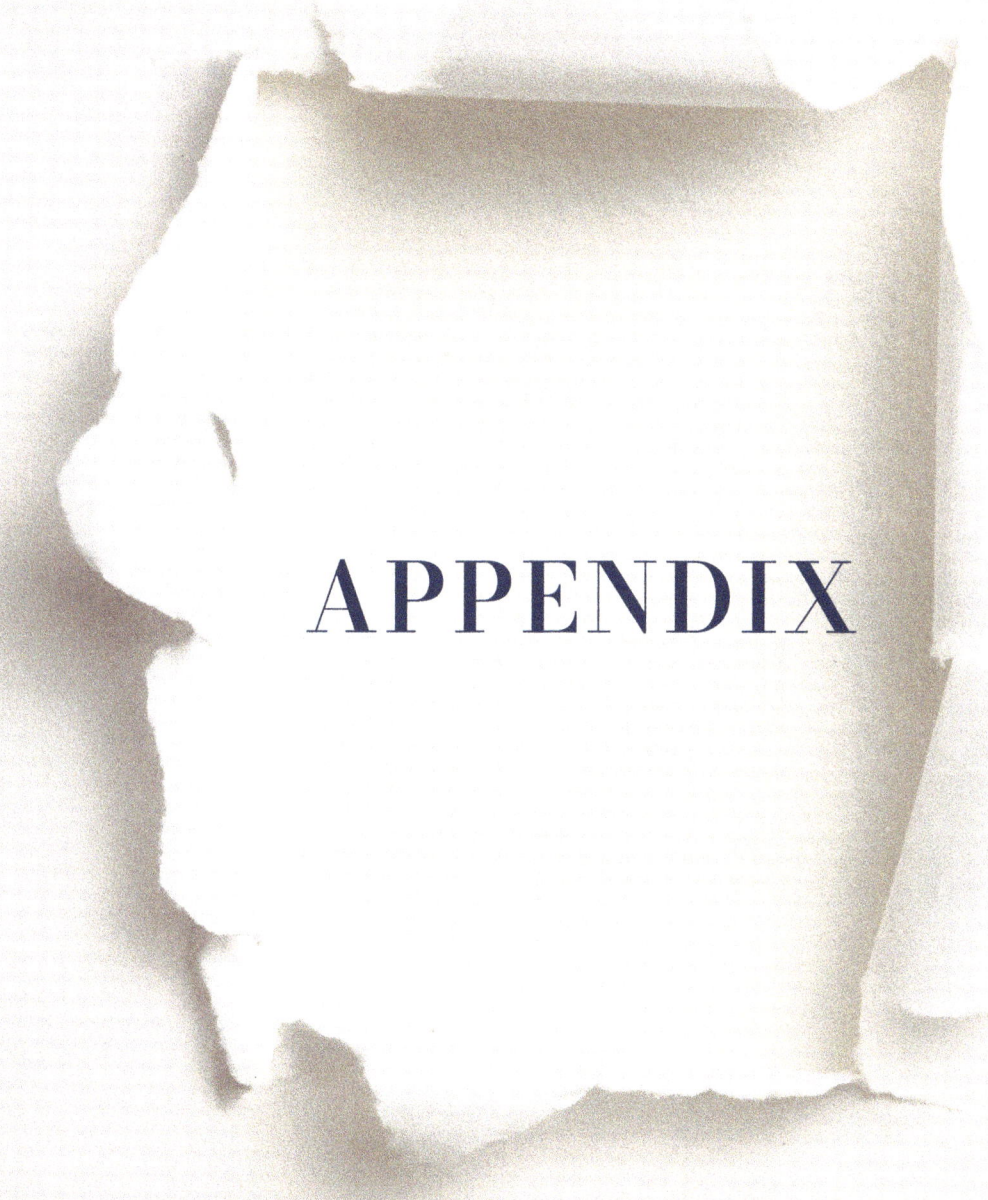

# APPENDIX

SUPERWELL

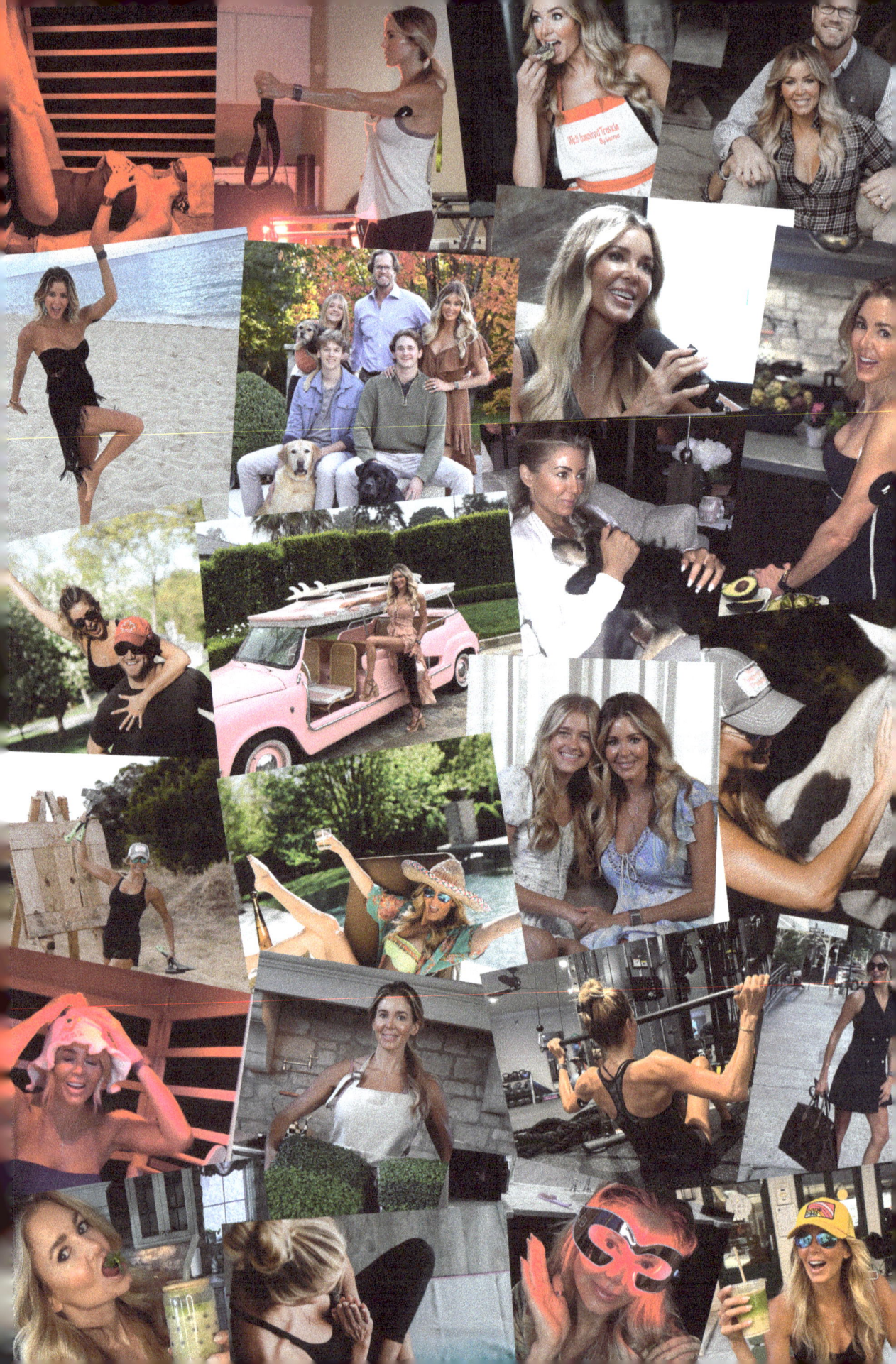

# MEET YOUR SUPERWELL-ISH LIVING BFF

**20 THINGS TO KNOW ABOUT LAUREN**

*(Because Besties Should Know Everything)*

1. I live for mornings. My day kicks off with grounding, red light, and my gut elixir in hand—dogs running around, barefoot on the grass, sunlight on my face. It's not a routine, it's my rhythm.

2. I believe laughter counts as core work. I've got a silly streak, a deep love for life, and if we're not belly-laughing at least once a day, what are we even doing?

3. Well Inspired Travels Founder: I launched Well Inspired Travels back in 2018 to blend my two obsessions—luxury travel and deep, soul-filling wellness. Think five-star stays with a side of transformation.

4. I'm a cold tub girlie. Yep, I sit in 40°F water and chat about real stuff—marriage, burnout, healing, growth. It's part therapy, part freeze-your-butt-off empowerment.

5. I don't fear sweat—I fear stagnation. I lift weights, stretch like a pretzel (triple-jointed, thanks Dad), and practice Pilates like it's a secret to life. Because it is.

6. I'm obsessed with red light therapy, protein shakes, and real conversations. Bonus points if we do all three at the same time.

7. My kids are my everything. They're my why, my greatest teachers, and the reason I show up in every part of my life with intention, fire, and love.

8. I keep it real. If you want the truth with a warm hug and a dash of sparkle—I'm your girl. I don't sugarcoat, but I do show up with compassion.

9. Peanut (my dog) is immortal. No, really. She's part soul guardian, part rescue pup, part boss of the house. If you know, you know.

10. I love a good glam moment, but I also live in my nerd bun. I can go from podcast-hosting wellness geek to full glam in 15 minutes flat. It's called balance.

11. Matcha > coffee. I traded cortisol crashes for calm energy. I froth mine with creatine and vanilla protein. Trust me, it's a vibe.

12. I make a killer 12-ingredient protein shake. It's kind of famous in my house. It fuels my day, supports my skin, and keeps my blood sugar in check. Basically, it's a hug in a glass (page 130).

13. Heat + cold is my love language. Contrast therapy reminds me that the most powerful breakthroughs happen just outside the comfort zone.

14. Meditation changed my life. Twice a day, I unplug to reset and refocus. I love sharing calming tools that help people breathe deeper, quiet the noise, and reconnect with themselves.

15. I'm the friend who reads ingredient labels. But I'll still split fries with you. Wellness isn't about rules—it's about rhythm, awareness, and living fully.

16. I've secretly matched eight couples. What can I say? I match people with soulmates and with spas. (Both require intuition and good vibes.)

17. I turned burnout into my blueprint. In 2011, everything in my life fell apart. I rebuilt it one habit at a time—and that's how SUPERWELL Living was born.

18. I biohack, but I don't overcomplicate. I track my glucose, wear red light masks, and love a good cold plunge—but I also believe in warm meals, naps, and sunshine.

19. I live for matcha mocktails, root veggie bowls, and sleep. Seriously, give me salmon, roasted beets, magnesium, and 8 hours in a cold bedroom, and I'm golden.

20. Best advice I ever got? Be yourself, fully. Your quirks are your magic. Your joy is your gift. Don't shrink—glow louder.

# ARE YOU READY TO STRIVE FOR SUPERWELL?

*Your journey doesn't end here.*

Scan the code below to access more resources like recipes, templates, and guides to help you continue thriving on your SUPERWELL path.

**SCAN FOR FREE ACCESS TO MORE RECIPES AND RESOURCES**

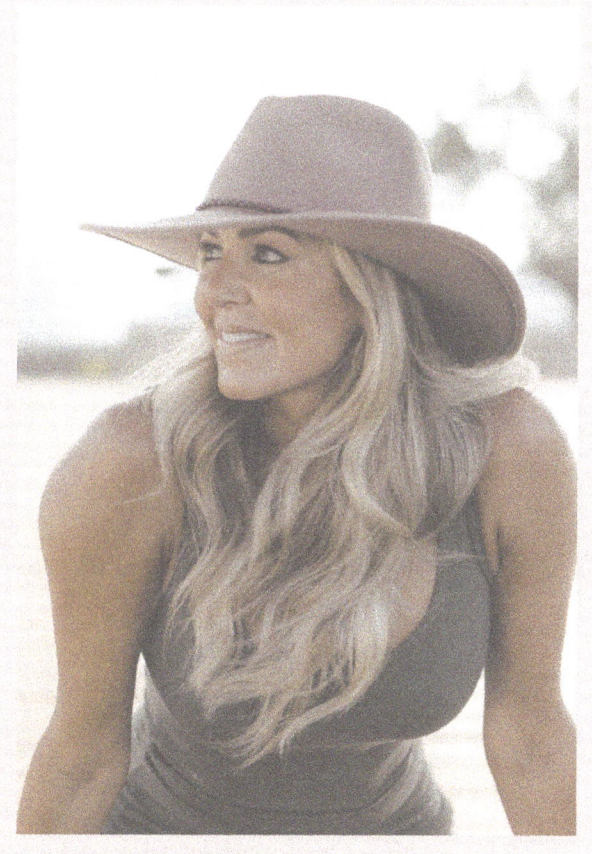

## WE ARE THE WELL STRIVING FOR SUPERWELL!

*Why the heck not?*

# SUPERWELL MANTRAS

- ✳ I'm in awe of how far I've come, and I'm just getting started.

- ✳ Nervous system regulation isn't just a goal—it's my grounding. I protect my peace like it's my job, because it is.

- ✳ My family is my home base. They're my why. My compass. My heart.

- ✳ True friendships are sacred. They hold me up, and I hold them just as high.

- ✳ Failure doesn't define me—it refines me. Every setback is a data point for growth.

- ✳ My boundaries are strong, loving, and rooted in self-respect. I honor them unapologetically.

- ✳ If it doesn't align with my energy, values, or heart—it's a no. Period.

- ✳ I'm flooded with gratitude every morning. Health, love, breath, purpose—I don't take it for granted.

- ✳ I've traded people-pleasing for self-trusting. My inner voice is my most loyal advisor.

- ✳ I welcome those who show up with love and integrity—and release those who don't with grace.

- ✳ Life is beautifully chaotic, and I've learned to ride the waves with strength, softness, and curiosity.

- ❋ My nervous system is my superpower. Breathwork, meditation, and stillness are non-negotiables.

- ❋ I no longer chase "skinny." I chase strong. I chase SUPERWELL.

- ❋ A walk in nature heals more than any scroll ever could.

- ❋ Nourishment comes before numbers. I fuel to feel.

- ❋ Meditation is my daily reset. Twenty minutes, twice a day—it's my gold.

- ❋ Mental health is foundational. I honor it like I do my physical body.

- ❋ Saying "no" when needed is my way of saying "yes" to myself.

- ❋ I let go often, forgive freely, and choose peace over pride.

- ❋ Humility is magnetic. It's what anchors me in truth and grace.

- ❋ I trust my intuition fiercely. She hasn't led me wrong yet.

- ❋ A kind gesture has the power to shift everything—and I lead with that intention.

- ❋ My evening routine is a love letter to my future self.

- ❋ Every day is a new chance to align my habits with my higher self.

- ❋ I am no longer chasing wellness. I am embodying SUPERWELL—one breath, one choice, one aligned moment at a time.

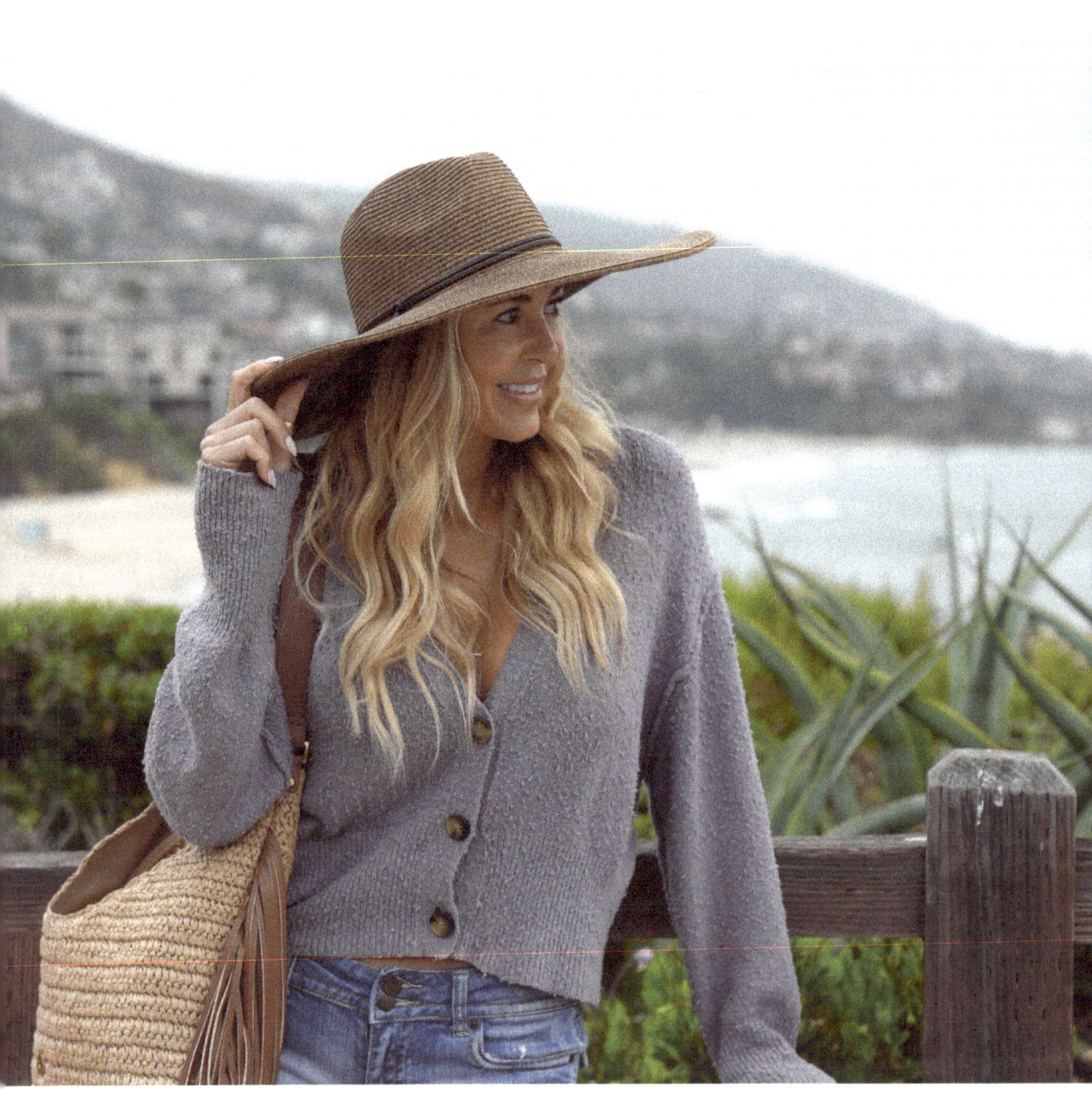

# YOUR SUPERWELL ALIGNMENT CHECK-INS

This is where transformation gets real—not in the rush, but in the rhythm. Whether you are closing out a season, reflecting on your month, or setting intentions for the week ahead, these check-ins are your personal space to pause, process, and recalibrate.

Each one is designed to reconnect you with your values, nervous system, and true self. Because living SUPERWELL isn't about perfection; it's about presence. It's about noticing what feels aligned, what needs support, and what deserves celebration.

Use these moments to shift from autopilot to intentionality. Let them be your grounding rituals in a world that rarely slows down. Tiny choices. Honest reflections. Big results.

Let's begin.

# SUPERWELL YEAR-END ALIGNMENT CHECK-IN

1. Where did I shift this year—mentally, emotionally, or spiritually?
   What belief, mindset, or pattern did I release or redefine that created realignment in my life?

2. What habits, people, or experiences made me feel most alive and regulated?
   Think energy-givers: Who or what helped elevate your nervous system and light you up from the inside out?

3. What drained my energy and pulled me out of alignment?
   What habits, obligations, or relationships left me feeling depleted, dysregulated, or out of touch with my authentic self?

4. Who were my *anchors* this year?
   Who grounded me when the seas of life felt choppy? Who held space for my growth, truth, and vulnerability?

5. Where did fear steer the ship instead of my intuition?
   What did I hold back on out of fear—fear of judgment, failure, or not being enough?

6. What were my most aligned wins, and where did I learn the most through challenge?
   Celebrate the highs, but honor the "misses" that became your greatest teachers.

7. What did life teach me this year about myself, others, and what truly matters?
   Where was the gold in the mess? What new awareness came forward?

8. What did I do that made me feel truly SUPERWELL?
   Think full mind-body-spirit alignment: What routines, trips, breakthroughs, or shifts supported you living in your highest vibration?

9. What areas of my life felt the most in flow, and which ones need some love?
   Where did ease exist? Where did resistance live? What's asking for more presence and nurturing

10. What are my top focuses for the year?
    Choose your 3–5 personal priorities for this next chapter:
    - Family & Parenting
    - Marriage or Partnership
    - Wellness & Recovery
    - Soulful Business Growth
    - Creative Expression
    - Nervous System Resilience
    - Exploration & Travel
    - Connection & Community

# SUPERWELL MONTHLY ALIGNMENT CHECK-IN

Because transformation happens in the tiny daily choices we repeat.

1. How did I support my nervous system this month?

   Did I practice breathwork, cold therapy, grounding, or create white space? Was I living in my sympathetic (stress) or parasympathetic (calm) state most of the time?

2. What habit stack worked beautifully, and which one needs a refresh?

   What part of my A.M. or P.M. ritual felt aligned, energizing, or effortless? What felt like a drag? What's one habit I could upgrade or remove?

3. What fueled me—literally and energetically?

   How did I nourish my body? Did I eat to feel strong and SUPERWELL? Which meals or supplements truly supported me? What needs adjusting?

4. What drained my energy or pulled me out of alignment?

   Was there a person, pattern, deadline, or thought loop? Did I spend too much time in tech noise, comparison, or caffeine-fueled chaos?

5. How did I invest in my inner world?

   Did I journal, meditate, walk in nature, or say "no" to protect peace? What did I do to connect with my higher self and values?

6. Did I rest, recover, and sleep well?

   Was I honoring my circadian rhythm? How was my sleep hygiene? How did I feel waking up most mornings—refreshed or depleted?

7. What boundaries felt empowering to hold? Which ones did I struggle with?

   Where did I overextend? Where did I reclaim my time and energy like a boss?

8. What was one moment that made me feel proud, grounded, or lit up this month?

   Big or small—what made me say "Yes. This is who I'm becoming."?

9. What do I want more of next month, and what needs to be lovingly released?

   More joy? More breath? Less noise? Less overthinking? Be honest and bold.

10. What's one non-negotiable SUPERWELL practice I'm committing to next month?

This could be 20 minutes of meditation, contrast therapy 3x/week, walking after meals, meal prepping on Sundays, or simply being present with your people.

# SUPERWELL SUNDAY SETUP

*Your Weekly Review to Reflect, Recalibrate, & Realign*

## 1. NERVOUS SYSTEM CHECK

- Where did I spend most of my time this week: regulated and calm, or stressed and reactive?
- What helped me shift into a parasympathetic state (breathwork, cold therapy, red light, meditation)?
- What were my stressors or triggers, and how did I respond?
- How can I support more calm and clarity this coming week?

## 2. WELLNESS WINS AND LESSONS

- What wellness habit served me best this week?
- Where did I fall short, without judgment?
- Was my movement intentional and supportive?
- Did I stay connected to my foundational practices like hydration, protein intake, contrast therapy, or sunlight?

## 3. SLEEP AND RECOVERY REFLECTION

- How many nights did I get high-quality sleep?
- What affected my HRV, deep sleep, or recovery markers?
- Did I shut down tech early, use red light, or support my sleep environment?
- How can I make sleep more of a sacred practice this week?

## 4. GUT AND BLOOD SUGAR AWARENESS

- Did I start the day with hydration and my gut elixir?
- What meals kept me balanced and energized?
- Did I experience crashes, bloating, or cravings that need attention?
- How can I better support my gut and glucose stability this week?

## 5. EMOTIONAL ENERGY INVENTORY

- What interactions or habits drained me?
- Who or what felt like a weight versus a lift?
- What boundaries need to be reinforced or redefined?
- Where did I feel aligned, light, and energized?

## 6. JOY AND ALIGNMENT CHECK

- What moments brought me real joy this week?
- Where did I feel most in my zone—connected, playful, or creative?
- How can I intentionally schedule more of that feeling this week?

## 7. RITUAL AUDIT: REPEAT, REFINE, OR RELEASE

- What should I repeat that worked beautifully?
- What needs a small adjustment to serve me better?
- What needs to be released for now—a habit, relationship, expectation, or task?

## 8. PLAN WITH ENERGY, NOT JUST TO-DO LISTS

- What are the most important commitments next week, and where do I need white space to reset?
- When will I move, meditate, recover, and recharge?
- Where does my calendar need breathing room?
- What is one personal or professional priority that matters most?

## 9. ENVIRONMENTAL AND LIFESTYLE SETUP

- Is my space clean, calm, and supporting my nervous system?
- Have I prepped meals, hydration tools, and wellness rituals for the week ahead?
- Are my clothes, journal, and red light set out for the morning?
- What small changes can I make to optimize my home, workspace, and sleep space?

## 10. WEEKLY ANCHOR WORD OR INTENTION

- Choose one word or intention to guide you this week. Examples: Clarity. Strength. Space. Peace. Focus. Grace. Nourishment. Boundaries. Write it down on a Post-it Note and stick it on your bathroom mirror to see each morning. Return to it each day.

# SUPERWELL
# MEDITATION MANTRAS

These meditation mantras were born from years of walking through burnout, healing my nervous system, and realigning my life from the inside out. They aren't just words; they are energetic resets. Anchors. Truths I return to when the world feels too loud, the schedule too full, or my inner peace starts to slip.

Whether you are carving out 20 minutes for stillness, walking through nature with your thoughts, or simply taking a breath between meetings or motherhood, let these mantras meet you where you are.

Pick the one that speaks to your soul and set the tone for your day. Let it ground you. Guide you. And gently remind you of the power you already hold within.

### FOR NERVOUS SYSTEM GROUNDING

- I am safe. I am steady. I am grounded in this moment.
- My breath is my anchor. I return to calm with every inhale and exhale.
- I live most powerfully when I live in peace.
- I am not the storm—I am the calm beneath it.

### FOR ENERGY AND VITALITY

- I radiate steady energy and vibrant health.
- My body is strong, my mind is focused, my spirit is alive.
- Every cell in my body is fueled with light and purpose.
- I choose habits that energize and elevate me.

## FOR SELF-WORTH AND CONFIDENCE

- I am more than enough just as I am
- My value is not up for debate. I embody strength and grace.
- I release comparison. I walk my own path with confidence.
- I don't shrink to fit spaces—I expand and elevate them.

## FOR STRESS AND EMOTIONAL RELEASE

- I release what no longer serves me and make space for peace.
- I allow myself to feel, and I allow myself to let go.
- I soften into this moment. I am allowed to rest.
- Tension leaves my body. Peace takes its place.

## FOR ALIGNMENT AND PURPOSE

- I am in alignment with who I'm meant to be.
- I trust the timing of my life.
- Everything I need is already within me.
- My choices create the rhythm of my life.

## FOR SLEEP AND EVENING CALM

- I release the day and welcome rest.
- My mind is quiet. My body is ready to restore.
- I trust in the stillness. I sink into deep rest.
- With each breath, I drift closer to peace.

www.ingramcontent.com/pod-product-compliance
Lightning Source LLC
Chambersburg PA
CBHW042357030426
42337CB00030B/5130